THE ESSENTIAL

HERBS

HANDBOOK

MORE THAN 100 HERBS FOR WELL-BEING,

HEALING, AND HAPPINESS

LESLEY BREMNESS

DUNCAN BAIRD PUBLISHERS

LONDON

The Essential Herbs Handbook
Distributed in the USA and Canada by
Sterling Publishing Co., Inc.,
387 Park Avenue South
New York, NY 10016-8810

This edition first published in the UK
and USA in 2009 by
Duncan Baird Publishers Ltd
Castle House, 75–76 Wells Street
London W1T 3QH

Copyright © Duncan Baird
Publishers 2009
Text and garden design copyright
© Lesley Bremness 2009
Commissioned photography copyright
© Duncan Baird Publishers 2009
For copyright of other photographs
see page 287, which is to be regarded
as an extension of this copyright.

The moral right of the author has
been asserted.

Consultant: Walter Enns

Library of Congress Cataloging-in-
Publication Data

Bremness, Lesley.
  The essential herbs handbook : more
than 100 herbs for well-being, healing,
and happiness / Lesley Bremness.
    p. cm.
  Includes bibliographical references
and index.
  ISBN 978-1-84483-801-1
  1. Herbs--Therapeutic use--Hand-
books, manuals, etc. I. Title.
  RM666.H33.B745 2009
  615'.321--dc22

                        2008046946

Printed in China by Imago

For information about custom editions,
special sales, premium and corporate
purchases, please contact Sterling
Special Sales Department at 800-805-
5489 or specialsales@sterlingpub.com.

Contents

Foreword

Turning to gardening was my instinctive response to years of city stress. In my tiny garden of the time, I decided on practicality over beauty and grew vegetables, but in my heart I wanted flowers. Then I discovered herbs: useful, beautiful plants that reconnect us with nature in profound ways.

I think of the study of herbs as a "gateway" subject. You might come to herbs because you have an interest in their flavours, but then you discover their nutritional benefits. Or perhaps you look into them so that you can make pure cosmetics, and then, unexpectedly, the world of herbal dyes opens up to you. As your matrix of connections grows, your relationship with nature deepens. When my own head seemed full of these connections, I started to write and teach about herbs so that I could share what I had learned.

After a few years my interest was drawn more toward the Taoist approach to nature – the more spiritual aspects of gardening – and I studied Chinese gardens. Writing this herbal has been an interesting journey back to herbs, and I am delighted by how much general understanding of these plants has expanded since I last focused on them. My initial enthusiasm for herbs has been re-ignited – and I can even glimpse a future in which scientists investigate the physics of herbs (at energetic and vibrational levels) to bring new insight into herbal–human interactions.

But with greater learning comes new fears about how we are treating our plants and planet. We must be the stewards of our local wild plants. If we want to make cowslip wine, we need to grow cowslips ourselves – in some countries it's illegal to pick those growing wild. Next, we must honour the herbalists throughout the world who have kept the knowledge of their herbs alive for thousands of years. If a company uses this local knowledge for profit, the local people should benefit. One worrying current trend is "biopiracy", where multinationals have managed to get patents on plant parts, and may attempt to exclude local people from selling their own plant products.

Working on this book has had one further, final gem to offer me. I have become more aware of the power of herbs not only to cure the body, but also to balance the mind and work with the subtleties of the spirit. I hope you enjoy discovering these remarkable gifts of nature as much as I have.

Safety – using herbs responsibly

- Never exceed the recommended dosages, and if you have concerns about amounts or the suitability of a herb, consult a professional herbalist.
- Generally, take remedies until your symptoms have gone. If there is no improvement within two to three weeks, see a professional practitioner.
- If you are taking conventional medicines or have planned surgery, tell your doctor you are taking herbal remedies and follow his or her advice.
- People aged over 70 should halve the recommended dosages. Consult a herbalist before giving herbal remedies to a child under age 12.
- If you are pregnant: avoid all herbal remedies during the first three months; avoid alcoholic tinctures throughout your pregnancy; and check individual entries for herbs that are specifically contraindicated for pregnant women.
- Never pick wild plants – grow the herbs you need yourself.
- If purchasing ready-prepared herbs, buy the best quality you can afford and always choose herbs from a reputable company.

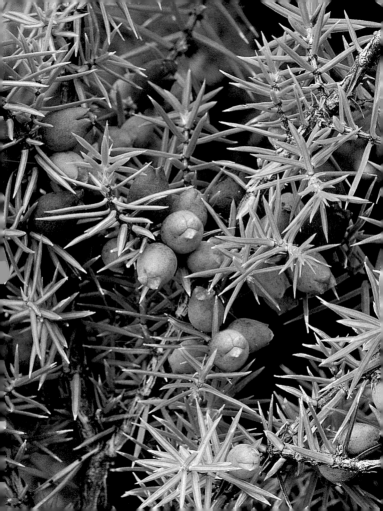

Part One:
The World of Herbs

Herbs are remarkable plants that touch every aspect of our lives: they reach us through our senses, they connect us with our ancestors and the world around us, and they enhance our physical, mental and spiritual well-being. In this section the world of herbs opens up to you. Discover what herbs are; track their history; unveil their importance in food, drinks, natural cosmetics, household fragrances and, above all, healing. Discover essential oils and flower essences and learn how to make herbal preparations so you have the confidence to use herbs for therapeutic value. And there is information on how to grow and harvest herbs, too, with suggestions for creating a herb garden – your own little corner of heaven.

What is a herb?

A herb is a plant that enriches our lives – as a food flavouring, a medicine, an object of meditation (through scent or appearance) or an ingredient in cosmetics and perfumes. Our assumptions about what a herb is mirror our cultural relationship with nature. At certain times in history, virtually all plants were considered herbs: in 1640, the English herbalist John Parkinson published his *Theatrum Botanicum*, which included botanical and medicinal information on a remarkable 3,800 plants. By the 20th century, the West's connection with nature had diminished so radically that many people knew of maybe a dozen or so herbs, and the term herb became common only for something we use as culinary seasoning. Fortunately, a recent cultural shift toward holistic healthcare means that we are revisiting more natural forms of medicine and our definition of a herb is expanding again.

Herbs for healing

Herbs are a cultural concept rather than a botanical definition, so healing herbs can come from any plant type (see opposite). The simple solutions to many of life's afflictions – such as stress, ill health and poor skin – often exist around us, in our gardens and woodlands. For example, to discover the blood-cleansing properties of an irritating weed such as burdock (see p.174) is a revelation. And now that we have access to the healing systems of other cultures, including those of China, India and ancient Persia, we've come to understand that many of the world's herbs can bring not only health and vitality to the body and mind, but harmony to the spirit, too. A herb can heal us on every level, because it brings nature back into our everyday lives.

Types of herbs

- **Trees:** Woody perennials (see below) with a single main trunk, from which branches grow usually well above ground to form a crown.

- **Shrubs:** Woody perennials (see below) with several, permanent woody stems (but no trunk) that grow from ground level. A shrub is usually smaller than a tree.

- **Perennials:** Non-woody plants that die back to roots in autumn, grow new shoots in spring and live for more than two growing seasons.

- **Biennials:** Plants that complete their life cycle over the course of two years. All biennials germinate and grow leaves in the first year and then flower and seed in the second.

- **Annuals:** Plants that complete their life cycle (from germination to bearing seeds, and then dying) in one growing season.

- **Vines and climbers:** Plants that have long, flexible stems and that climb up, twine around or apply tendrils or suckers to other, sturdier plants or to objects, for support.

- **Fungi:** Plants, commonly called mushrooms, with a domed cap-like body. On the underside of the cap are gills that produce a huge number of spores, which the plant releases once they are mature.

11

Herbs through history

People have relied upon herbs to please their stomachs, to heal their bodies and to connect with their gods as long as we have been on this planet – herb seeds have been found in archaeological sites dating back 200,000 years. Early humans selected and used herbs by observing the plants that animals ate, through inspiration and creative thought, and by trial and error. Over time, oral tradition enabled an accumulated knowledge of herbs to pass down through generations. Gradually, humankind refined its understanding of plants to give us the complex systems of herbalism we have today.

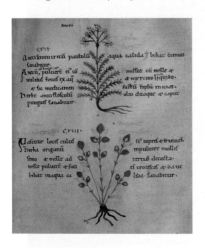

Ancient beginnings

One widespread early use of herbs seems to have been in ritual and magic. In belief systems throughout the world, the concept of the spirit realm was closely linked with all levels of human well-being, and herbs provided a bridge between earthly existence and spiritual or higher nature. As human thought

The *Bury St Edmunds Herbal* (c.1120) is noted for its naturalistic illustrations of several of the herbs it features.

became more sophisticated, early beliefs evolved into holistic healing systems incorporating body, mind and spirit. The most notable are Indian Ayurvedic medicine (see pp.16–17) and Traditional Chinese Medicine (see pp.18–19).

In Tibet, Australia and the Americas, indigenous peoples drew upon their intimate relationship with nature for ways to use healing herbs in ritual and medicine. In Australia, the Aborigines' experience with herbs such as eucalyptus (which aids breathing) and tea tree (a natural antiseptic) has led us to value these herbs highly, too. Native North American healers "listened" to the plants. Their knowledge has taught us about the powers of echinacea (p.98), sagebrush (p.256) and juniper (p.266), among many others.

However, it is in Africa that we find the most ancient and diverse herbal traditions. In every corner of this vast continent, herbal systems, even today, pervade all aspects of medicine – indeed, in remote areas herbs may provide the only treatments available. Around 1,550BCE, in northern Africa, the ancient Egyptians produced the *Ebers Papyrus*, a scroll of 811 herbal prescriptions that encouraged physicians to address all levels of being in order to cure the "whole" person. Two hundred years later, this document inspired the legendary Greek healer Asclepius to set up his own healing centres, where he made significant use of herbs to purge and cleanse mind, body and spirit.

From spirit to science

Asclepius's healing system attracted many followers, one of whom was Hippocrates (460–377BCE), who dismissed the early idea that magic or demons caused illness and instead based his practice on observation.

He stated firmly that the body must be treated as a whole, and included diet, fresh air, hygiene and rest with his herbal treatments.

Around 175CE, the Greek physician Galen further codified Hippocrates' ideas, and in doing so formed a basis for European medicine that would last for 1,500 years. Eventually, however, the Roman "mechanistic" view of the body – which considered and treated body parts separately – was reinforced by pharmaceutical science. This marginalized the holistic approach, and herbal medicine, with its roots in nature, fell out of fashion.

The rebirth of herbalism

For centuries, herbalism was kept alive by local herb women, and by monks, who use herbs in monastic activities such as brewing and soap-making. But then came the Renaissance – a time for re-examining old ideas, and of breaking free from dogma to pursue new discoveries. Herbalism returned to fashion and scientists looked at remedies with refreshingly open minds, assessing efficacy and cataloguing treatments with new accuracy.

Then, in the 15th century, the invention of the printing press transformed people's access to knowledge. An understanding of herbs that had once been solely the province of medics and monks, became available to all in the form of medicinal herbals (see box, opposite). Strangely, though, in this environment of progressive thought, there were also cruel witch hunts, often against women herbalists. Women were forbidden to study and non-professional healers were open to accusations of heresy. Influenced by these attitudes, some people continue to equate herbalism with superstition and quackery.

Herbalism and modern medicine

Even for those who are sceptical about the relevance of herbalism in treating disease, it is undeniable that many modern pharmaceuticals derive from herbs. Take Aspirin™. This everyday painkiller is made using salicylic acid, a compound isolated from meadowsweet and willow. However, when active ingredients are isolated, any modulators (perhaps against side-effects) or enhancers that exist naturally in the plant are lost. It is often better to take a herb, with all its properties, than to take a medicine with only one.

This, and a feeling that pharmaceuticals contain too many toxins, is turning many of us back to natural medicine. Research around the world is validating – and making exciting new discoveries about – the medicinal uses of plants. Science is coming full circle, and the future for herbs is brighter than ever.

The European herbals

One of the earliest European herbals is *De Materia Medica* (65CE) by the Roman army physician Dioscorides. For almost 2,000 years, this provided an invaluable resource on the botany and virtues of 600 herbs. Increasingly detailed works followed, by writers such as the German abbess Hildegard of Bingen (1098–1179), the Swiss physician Paracelsus (1493–1541) and the 16th- and 17th-century English botanists William Turner, John Gerard and John Parkinson. In 1653, another Englishman, Nicholas Culpeper, published his *Complete Herbal*, a work containing 394 herbs, which, still in print 350 years later, is arguably the most popular herbal of all time.

Herbs in Ayurveda

The Indian word *ayurveda*, meaning the "science of life", is the name given to India's 4,000-year-old system of holistic healthcare. Ayurveda treats the body, mind and spirit through such disciplines as diet, yoga and meditation, and also through the use of herbs. Ginger (see p.68), brahmi (p.74), neem (p.118), ashwagandha (p.250) and sandalwood (p.274) – among thousands of others – are all herbs with noble histories in Ayurvedic medicine.

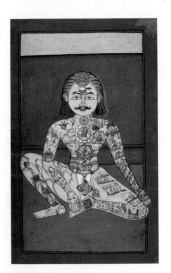

The three *doshas*

In Ayurveda, all matter is composed of five elements: space, air, fire, water and earth. There are three physical body types or *doshas*: *vata* (influenced by air and space); *pitta* (fire and water); and *kapha* (water and earth). Each of us has one dominant *dosha*, which, when we are ill, an Ayurvedic physician will take into account before creating a remedy that may contain up to 25 healing herbs.

An 18th-century illustration of the seven *chakras* placed vertically down the mid-line of the body, from crown to root.

Herbs and the *chakras*

Western herbalists suggest herbs to influence the body's main *chakras* – seven spinning wheels of energy (listed below) linking our physical, emotional, mental and spiritual levels with life energy (*prana*). *Chakras* reflect spiritual growth; when we use herbs to help balance the *chakra* areas, it is easier for our spirit to unfold.

- **Crown *chakra*** (top of the head) – this is the *chakra* of spiritual integration. The herbs nutmeg (p.60), gotu kola (p.76) and valerian (p.220) influence it.

- **Third eye or brow *chakra*** (on the brow) – the *chakra* of clarity and inner vision, it is balanced by basil (p.82), blue skullcap (p.216) and sandalwood (p.274).

- **Throat *chakra*** (at the throat) – this *chakra* governs our communication powers and is balanced by clove (p.64), licorice (p.100) and frankincense (p.258).

- **Heart *chakra*** (on the breastbone) – this is the *chakra* of love, and responds to the energies of saffron (p.228) and rose (p.242).

- **Solar plexus *chakra*** (at the navel) – governing personal strength, this *chakra* is influenced by black pepper (p.84), goldenseal (p.102) and oregano (p.104).

- **Sacral *chakra*** (just below the navel) – this *chakra* is the hub of our creative and sexual energy. Fennel (p.122) and coriander (p.226) are its balancing herbs.

- **Root *chakra*** (at the base of the spine) – this *chakra* is the home of the first movement of energy, our motivation. Its balancing herb is ashwagandha (p.250).

Herbs in Traditional Chinese Medicine

Traditional Chinese Medicine (TCM) originated as part of the Taoist philosophy, which evolved in China around 4,500 years ago. When treating patients, as well as drawing upon practices such as massage, exercise and meditation, TCM practitioners call upon a treasure chest of over 2,000 herbs.

Healing energies

In Taoism, all the world's phenomena, from the stars to a flea, result from the interplay of opposite forces – of *yin* (which is dark, cool, moist, inward) and *yang* (bright, hot, dry, outward) – as they create a continuous spiral of change. The Taoist Masters ate particular herbs to feel their *yin* or *yang* effect. Sage (p.164) is a cooling *yin* tonic; ginger (p.68) is a warming *yang* herb. In addition, each herb is assigned one of five "tastes" (bitter, sweet, pungent, salty or sour), which themselves represent one of the Five Elements (fire, earth, metal, water and wood) that connect humanity with nature.

Taoists describe their own body energies in terms of three types. These are the Three Treasures, *jing*, *chi* and *shen*. *Jing* is the inherited nutritive essence, nurtured by food and herbs, but drained by stress. Stress-busting herbs such as dang shen (p.140) and ginseng (p.158) help restore *jing*. *Chi* (sometimes written *qi*) is the life force that flows along energy pathways, called meridians, in the body. When the life force is free-flowing, we experience wellness. Licorice (p.100) is taken to allow *chi* to flow smoothly. *Shen* is our spiritual energy, which brings higher consciousness. The legendary reishi mushroom (p.148) is taken as the "herb of spiritual potency". Practitioners particularly value schisandra (p.108), because it enhances all the Three Treasures.

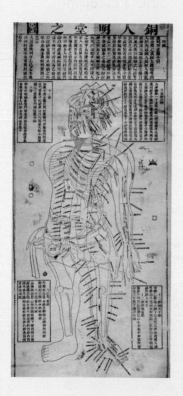

Diagnosis and treatment

TCM is a holistic approach, because it considers the *yin–yang*, the Five Elements, and the *jing*, *chi* and *shen* energies of a patient, as well as his or her pulse and breath, and tongue and skin health. Practitioners know that a virus causes a cold, but they aim to correct the imbalance that let the virus invade in the first place.

Most treatments use a combination of herbs, from groups called "kingly", "ministerial", "servant" and "slave". The most highly valued are the kingly herbs, such as ginseng, astragalus (p.96) and licorice, which harmonize all the body's systems and boost immunity to create the best platform for self-healing.

This 19th-century Chinese illustration shows the meridian lines, through which energy must flow freely for good health.

Herbal preparations

Herbal preparations enable us to take or apply herbs therapeutically. They may be internal, such as an infusion or decoction, or external, as in a compress or poultice. Each of the herbs in the Guide (see pp.46–275) has a preparations panel suggesting how to make your remedies for the best therapeutic value. Use the quantities in the panel; then, when advised, refer to the instructions below for the standard method on how to make the preparation.

Internal preparations

Infusion: Brewed like tea, an infusion is used for delicate leaves and flowers. Steep the recommended quantity in 1 cup of just-boiled water for 10 minutes (this makes one dose). Strain before drinking, or leave the herbs as sprigs and simply remove them. Always cover infusions if you intend to store them, and use them within 24 hours. Drink hot or cold.

Decoction: This method is used for tougher plant parts, such as bark, roots and some berries. Place the relevant quantity of herbs in 750ml (1½ pints) cold water (makes three doses) in a Pyrex® or enamel pot. Boil, then simmer for 1 hour to reduce the liquid by a third. Strain through a nylon sieve into a jug and store, covered, in a cool place for up to 24 hours. Drink hot or cold.

Tincture: To make a tincture, a herb is steeped in an alcohol, such as vodka, to extract the active ingredients. Place the recommended quantity of herb in a clean glass jar and add 1 litre (2 pints) of a vodka-water mix (use ²/₃ vodka to ¹/₃ water), ensuring that you cover the herbs. Seal the jar and shake well. Put it in a cool, dark place for two weeks, shaking daily. After this, strain the liquid by squeezing it through muslin, and rebottle (it will last for two years). Dilute each recommended dosage in 30ml (1fl oz) water or juice before drinking.

Capsule: If you are taking a bitter or spicy herb, such as cayenne (see p.50), you may prefer it in capsule form. Filling your own capsules ensures that you avoid any fillers, binders or preservatives. Buy size 00 gelatine or vegetarian

When making infusions, always use a teapot or cup with a lid. Keep the lid on as the herbs are steeping in order to prevent volatile oils (part of the active ingredients) evaporating.

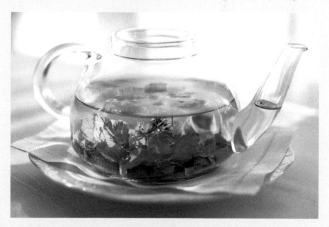

capsules and the relevant herb powder. Place a little powder in a saucer and scoop it into the two halves of the capsule to fill them; push them together. One capsule will hold 500mg of powder. You can store your capsules in a labelled, airtight, dark-glass bottle in a cool place for four months.

Tonic wine: This is a pleasant way to take digestive or tonic herbs. Put the suggested quantity of herb in a large glass or ceramic jar with 1 litre (2 pints) of red or white wine (red is best). Stir well and replace the lid. Leave to mature for two to six weeks (the longer the better), then strain. Discard if mould develops.

External preparations

Steam inhalation: A steam inhalation is a wonderful way to relieve congestion (used as a facial steam, it will also cleanse the skin; see p.24).

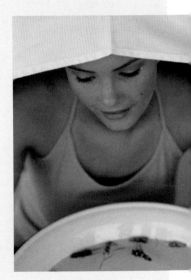

Inhaling herb-infused steam allows the herb's beneficial properties direct access to the lungs, and to the pores of the skin.

Place 2 handfuls fresh herbs or 3 tbsp dried herbs in a bowl. Pour over 1.5 litres (3 pints) boiling water, then stir. Lean over the bowl, using a towel to make a tent that covers both your head and the bowl. Close your eyes and, if this is not uncomfortable, stay there, breathing gently, for 10 to 15 minutes.

Poultice: Apply a poultice to relieve soreness and inflammation of the skin. Add very hot water to herb powder to make a paste, or simmer sufficient chopped fresh or dried herb to cover the area in a little water for 2 minutes, then squeeze out the water. Spread the powder or fresh-herb paste over your skin as hot as you can tolerate and bandage it in place with gauze. Leave it there for two to three hours, then repeat if necessary.

Compress: A hot compress is another great way to reduce inflammation or ease skin irritation and is less messy than a poultice. Soak a gauze, cotton or linen cloth in the strength of infusion or decoction recommended in the Guide. Then squeeze out the excess liquid, fold the cloth and hold it against the skin. Repeat the process when the compress cools or dries, as required.

Infused oil: This will lubricate the skin for massage. Fill a clean glass jar with fresh leaves or flowers, then pour in olive oil to cover the herbs. Leave the jar on a sunny windowsill for two to three weeks, stirring occasionally. Pour the mix into a suspended muslin bag to filter through to a bowl below. Squeeze out the remaining oil. Repeat the process using the same oil but fresh herbs for a stronger infused oil. Store in dark-glass bottles for six to 12 months.

Cosmetic uses for herbs

In a world full of toxins, making your own cosmetic products is the only way to guarantee the purity and freshness of the ingredients you put on your skin.

Cleansing creams, moisturizers, tonics, face packs, herbal soaps, and hand-, foot-, nail- and hair-care products can all be made at home. Several simple recipes are found under individual herbs in the Guide (see, for example, the elderflower cream for chapped skin on page 107 or the calendula ointment on page 121). In addition, two of the simplest – but loveliest – ways to enjoy the benefits of herbs, and do wonders for your skin at the same time, are facial steams and herbal baths.

Facial steams

A facial steam provides a thorough, deep cleanse of the skin. The heat makes the skin gently perspire, eliminating toxins and freeing up the circulation; while the steam softens the skin and opens the pores to absorb the properties of the herbs. Before you have your steam, tie back your hair and gently cleanse your face using your usual cleanser. Follow the steam inhalation instructions on page 22. For normal skin use stinging nettle (p.190), lavender (p.202) or German chamomile (p.204); for oily skin, calendula (p.120), sage (p.164) or yarrow (p.170); for dry skin, lady's mantle (p.114), sweet violet flowers and leaves (p.134), parsley (p.180) or borage (p.198); and for mature or sallow skin, elderflower (p.106), dandelion (p.186), or red clover flowers and leaves (p.188). Once you've finished, rinse your face with tepid water, and again five minutes later with cold. To tighten your pores, dab on an infusion or diluted herb vinegar (see p.32) of elderflower, peppermint (p.58), sage or yarrow.

Herbal baths

A herbal bath can help rejuvenate the skin and heal the body. To stimulate your circulation, try herbs such as bay (p.80), basil (p.82) or fennel (p.122). To soothe aching muscles, add rosemary (p.86). If you need to relax and unwind, try any of the relaxing herbs on pages 194–220. Or, choose a herb for its particular healing properties.

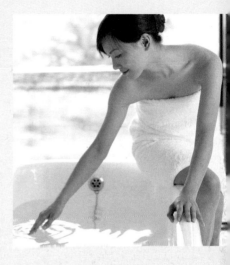

Place a handful of herbs in a muslin bag, secure the top and leave the bag in the water. As an alternative, if you prefer, you can swirl 1 litre (2 pints) of an infusion or a decoction (see p.20) into the bath water. Relax in the warm (but not hot) water for at least 10 minutes.

To ease itchy skin or aching muscles, try a herbal vinegar bath. Add 500ml (1 pint) herb-infused cider vinegar (see p.32) to the water. Or to soften and soothe skin, have a milk bath. Put 3 tbsp powdered whole milk in a muslin bag with a handful of fresh elderflowers (p.106), chamomile flowers (p.204) or lime blossoms (p.218). Swish the closed bag around in the water as you bathe. 25

Using essential oils

An essential oil is the concentrated aromatic essence of a fragrant plant. The oil exists in special cells in the plant's flowers, leaves, seeds, peel, wood, resin and/or roots. We know of more than 400 plant essences that we can extract, and around 100 of these are currently available for us to buy.

An essence gives a plant its flavour and contributes to its therapeutic value (in the plant itself, the essence provides antiseptic protection, perhaps even defending it against fungi and viruses), but it is its fragrance that has the greatest appeal. Inhaling the scent from these aromatic molecules has instant effects on our mind, body and spirit: an essential oil can be uplifting, calming or energizing, or may bring about a sense of spiritual transformation.

Capturing fragrance

The reason we are able to smell something – whether it's a flower, a leaf, or a certain food – is because that item's aromatic molecules continually bounce into the air. When we inhale, the bouncing molecules touch the scent organ at the back of our nose and trigger an electrical pulse that goes directly to our brain. This is why scent is so immediately evocative – think how certain smells can instantly spark the recall of memories, even those buried deep within you.

We can capture these aromatic molecules in infused oils (see p.23) and alcohols (see p.20), but also in skin lotions – for example, we could add fresh jasmine petals to an unscented face cream to give it both the fragrance and the skin benefits of the herb. In a bottle of essential oil, the work is done for you. Producers steam distil the aromatic plant parts (it takes the petals of 60,000 roses to create 30g/1oz rose oil) to condense then siphon off the oil.

Applying the oils

The most common use for essential oils is in aromatherapy: oils are diluted in a carrier oil, such as sweet almond, and applied to the body during massage. However, there are many other ways to use essential oils to improve well-being. I like to make room sprays to deodorize and refresh a room, deter insects, neutralize microbes and create a mood. There are many examples within the Guide – try a peppermint spray to refresh and re-energize (see p.59), or a clove spray to create an inviting sense of warmth (see p.65).

Staying safe

Essential oils are wonderful – but highly potent. Use only the recommended amounts and always dilute them in a carrier oil before putting them on your skin (a few drops of oil in a bathful of water is okay, too). Never take essential oils internally, and keep them away from your eyes. If you are pregnant, have sensitive skin, or suffer from any health complaint, consult an aromatherapist.

An essential-oil study aid

If you are studying for an exam, place a few drops of a clean-smelling essential oil (say, basil, rosemary or lemon) on the pages of your textbook to sniff as you revise (choose a different oil for each subject). Then, on the day of your exam, infuse a tissue with a few drops of that oil, put it in a plastic bag to keep it fresh, and take it into the exam with you to sniff periodically and spark the relevant memory area in your brain.

Domestic uses for herbs

Five hundred years ago, all aspects of domestic life would have involved the use of herbs. By revisiting some of these traditional methods, we can make our homes cleaner and fresher in ways that enhance our well-being – and, because they are completely safe, that protect our environment, too.

In your living space

The easiest way to bring herbs into your home is to put a few sprigs of something fresh and aromatic in a vase. Alecost, angelica, basil, bay, calendula, evening primrose, hyssop, juniper, lavender, lemon balm, peppermint, rosemary, sage, sweet cicely, sweet myrtle and thyme are all good choices as they will scent and purify the air. To the same end, keep unused prunings of lavender, rosemary, sage, thyme and juniper in a jar near the hearth to sprinkle on the fire – burning them will release their fragrance.

A vase or pot of lavender placed strategically on a windowsill or mantelpiece can lift your spirits each time you pass by.

Cinnamon and cloves sprinkled around books will protect them from pests and, in a home office, a dish of dried lavender flowers by the phone will relax you if you run your fingers through it while making stressful calls.

In your kitchen

To disguise cooking fumes, deter flies and freshen the air, make a dish of kitchen pot pourri. Use dried herbs in the following quantities: 1 part lemon and 1 part orange peel; 2 parts peppermint, 2 parts bay, 1 part basil, 1 part neem leaves; and 1 part chamomile flowers and a few crushed cloves. Then, to clean your kitchen, put three handfuls of fresh or dried rosemary, thyme and oregano in 4 cups water in a pan and simmer with the lid on for 15 minutes, then strain. Use the liquid as an antiseptic wash for your surfaces.

In your bedroom

Fragrant, antiseptic herbs can improve your sleep (try the bay sleep cushion on page 80) and sweeten the scent of stored clothes and protect them from moths. Lay small cotton bags of aromatic herbs among the clothes in your drawers. Alecost, lavender, rosemary, angelica and neem are all good choices.

In your garden

You can use herbs to make your own, natural fertilizer – try the method using comfrey on page 127 (you could use nettle leaves, too). If you have a compost heap, a few chopped yarrow leaves sprinkled between the layers of compost will help speed up decomposition.

Purifying household air

As many synthetic building materials, paints, treated woods, cleaning agents and furniture polishes give off potentially harmful chemicals in our homes, we can be assaulted on all sides by small but cumulative amounts of toxins. Add to this cocktail dry air and unventilated spaces from tightly sealed buildings and it's easy to see how we can become ill. In work spaces, when staff develop symptoms such as skin rashes, itchy eyes and nasal allergies, plus vague problems such as aches and pains, fatigue and odour sensitivity, poor air quality is often to blame. This is known as "sick building syndrome".

Help from NASA and beyond

Fortunately for us, NASA (the North American Space Agency) considered this syndrome a potential problem for space stations and has now identified 50 houseplants that remove various gases and pollutants from interiors. The top ten are: the heartleaf philodendron (*Philodendron scandens* 'oxycardium'), the elephant ear philodendron (*Philodendron domesticum*), cornstalk dracaens (*Dracaena fragrans* 'Massangeana'), English ivy (*Hedera helix*), the spider plant (*Chlorophytum comosum*), the Janet Craig dracaena (*Dracaena deremensis* 'Janet Craig'), the Warneck dracaena (*Dracaena deremensis* 'Warneckii'), the weeping fig (*Ficus benjamina*), golden pothos (*Epipiremnum aureum*) and the peace lily (*Spathiphyllum* 'Mauna Loa').

On the New York Stock Exchange, concern about computer emissions has led workers to purify their space with the Peruvian cactus (*Cereus uruguayanus*). Not only does this plant have beautiful white, scented flowers, it appears to reduce the electromagnetic pollution emitted by office hardware.

Putting it into practice

As a general rule grow one plant per 9m² (100 sq ft) of floor space. Where possible, group plants together in trays of gravel, and add rosemary, thyme or lavender, as they tolerate dry air and can release antiseptic essential oils. As well as absorbing air pollutants, groups of plants bring a window of stress-reducing nature inside and boost levels of fresh oxygen in enclosed spaces.

When NASA tested houseplants for their ability to remove formaldehyde from a gas chamber, the spider plant (*Chlorophytum comosum*) removed 95 percent of the toxic gas in just 24 hours.

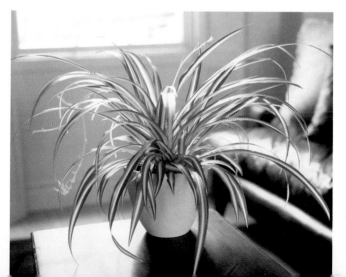

Nutrition and flavour

One of the most pleasurable ways to benefit from herbs is in food. Herbs transform a dish into an aromatic experience; moreover, packed with vitamins, minerals and trace elements, each herb contributes to nutritional well-being. Use fresh herbs in your cooking, or capture a herb's flavour, and many of its therapeutic properties, by preserving and using it in the following ways.

Herb vinegars: Bruise freshly picked leaves or seeds and loosely fill a clean glass jar. Pour over warmed (not hot) cider or wine vinegar to cover, and place on a sunny windowsill, shaking daily for two weeks. For a stronger vinegar, strain and repeat with fresh herbs. Store as it is, or strain through muslin and then rebottle. Add a fresh sprig of the herb for identification.

Flower vinegars: These are made in the same way as herb vinegars. Try the flowers of clover, elder, lavender, orange or rose. Use these vinegars in tiny amounts to add an aromatic twist to fruit dishes, such as fruit salad.

Herb oils: Culinary herb oils are made in the same way as the infused oil on page 23, using any mild-flavoured cooking oil, such as sunflower. Try infusing basil, garlic, fennel, oregano, mint, rosemary or thyme to use in salad dressings and marinades, or for softening vegetables and browning meat.

Basil, bay, dill, garlic, fennel, lemon balm, oregano, mint, rosemary, thyme, or combinations of any of these, make wonderful herb vinegars to use in salad dressings, marinades, sauces and gravies. Try purple fennel, too, which turns a clear vinegar a beautiful ruby-red.

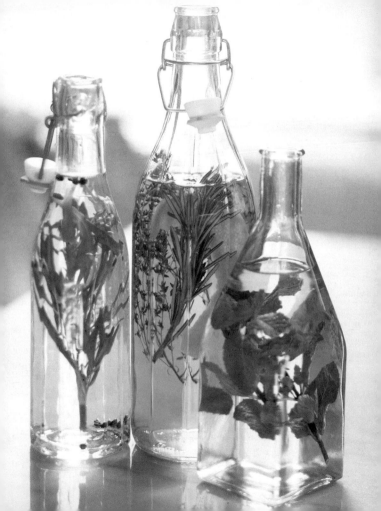

Flower essences

Flower essences heal at a purely energetic level, correcting imbalances in the human spirit and emotions. They were made famous by Dr Edward Bach, who in the 1930s gave up his lucrative London medical practice to heal patients through nature. The principle is that every flower has a unique vibrational pattern of healing energy, which can be transferred to water, via sunlight.

Throughout the Guide, I have recommended flower essences for spiritual growth. However, my suggestions are only to steer you: selecting a flower essence should itself be a process of inner growth – something led by intuition. If you are making flower essences (see opposite), choose a time when both you and the environment around you feel positive and peaceful.

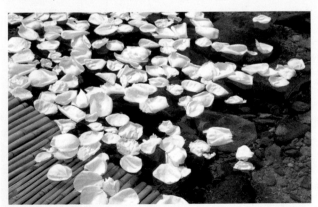

Making a flower essence

1 Find a glass plate, a pair of scissors, tweezers, a 2-litre (4-pint) glass bowl, 1 litre (2 pints) pure water, and two 1-litre (2-pint) lidded glass jars, half-filled with brandy.

2 Sterilize your equipment in hot, soapy water and rinse well. Avoid touching the inside of the bowl once it is cleaned.

3 Choose a sunny morning and wait until the dew has gone. Approach your chosen plant with respect, and meditate to connect with its life force.

4 Select flowers (usually up to five of them) that are a day from being completely opened. Snip the heads onto the glass plate, taking care not to touch or sniff them.

5 Fill the glass bowl with the pure water and place it in the sun, preferably next to the contributing plant.

6 Remove the petals, using the scissors or tweezers (not your fingers), gently shaking off any stamens or insects, and place them individually in the bowl of water.

7 Meditate with the spirit of the plant for one minute, to request that the healing properties of the flowers be transferred by sunlight into the water. Then leave the bowl of petals in the sun for three hours to complete the transferring process.

8 Remove the petals from the bowl using tweezers and discard them; top up the half-filled brandy jars with the solarized flower solution. Secure the lids, label and date. This is your mother tincture and will keep for several years. To use it, dilute it into stock bottles: place 2 drops of mother tincture in a 30ml/1fl oz stock bottle and top up with brandy. (Stock-bottle strength is what you would buy in the shops.)

Dosage: Individual dosages are given in the Guide, but as a general rule put 2 drops flower essence from the stock bottle into a glass of water and sip throughout the day, or put 2 drops directly from the stock bottle under your tongue.

Planting a herb garden

Having your own herb garden gives you a chance to grow a collection of beautiful, evocative and useful plants with connections to all aspects of healthy living. You can grow herbs in vegetable or flower beds, in containers on balconies and patios, in window boxes, and even inside. As many herbs are wild species, they are easy to grow. The key is to find the right position, soil type, and where appropriate container size, for each plant.

Finding a site in a garden

To accommodate a wide range of herbs, choose a quiet, well-drained site with three-quarters of the area in sun most of the day. Partly enclose the space with a hedge or screen to create privacy, provide wind shelter (to contain fragrances and allow bees longer working hours), muffle sound and block unsightly views. Use this as an opportunity for creativity: give the hedge a curved top, or use willow screens that have a seat woven into one panel.

Making space for picking

If you are planting your herbs in the ground, for convenience make your soil beds a maximum 1.5m (5ft) wide, so you can reach easily to pick them. A path layout, whether formal or informal, is your next design element – with a hard surface to walk on, even in rain you will be able to nip out for a sprig of parsley or few leaves of basil. Think of the paths as part of the beauty of your herb garden – they can give decorative shapes, textures and colours all year round, even when seasonal plants have died away. Again, try to think creatively: use recycled materials and pebble designs to add interest.

Planting your herbs

Make a list of the herbs you'd like to plant, then check their hardiness and sun and soil needs in the Guide (pp.46–275). Position the herbs first for their sun and shade requirements, then by use – for example, put your salad herbs together. Allow roughly 10 plants per m² (or 1 plant per sq ft). If you are planting a herb that has been growing in a container, dig a hole greater than the pot size, place good compost in the bottom, and set the plant in the centre, filling in with new compost. Press the plant in gently and water well.

You don't need a huge garden to be able to grow herbs. A few pots and a small patio, sunny balcony or sturdy window box can provide ample space for your very own herbal sanctuary.

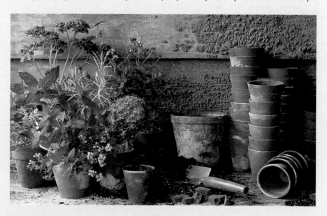

Patio, balcony or rooftop herb garden

This sample garden design would work well for a small patio, a roof garden or even a balcony. If you can, try to make space for seating – a place to rest and enjoy your special environment.

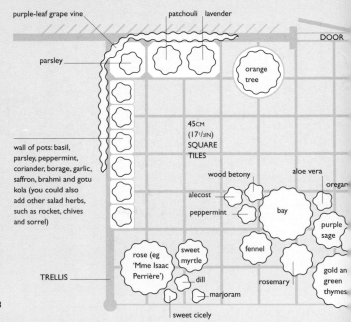

purple-leaf grape vine

patchouli lavender

DOOR

parsley

orange tree

45CM
(17¹/₂IN)
SQUARE
TILES

wall of pots: basil, parsley, peppermint, coriander, borage, garlic, saffron, brahmi and gotu kola (you could also add other salad herbs, such as rocket, chives and sorrel)

wood betony

aloe vera

oregan

alecost

peppermint

bay

purple sage

rose (eg 'Mme Isaac Perrière')

sweet myrtle

fennel

gold an green thymes

TRELLIS

dill

rosemary

marjoram

sweet cicely

38

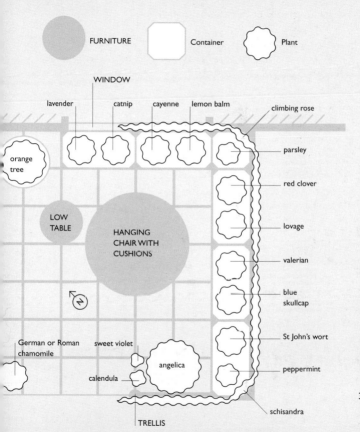

FURNITURE

Container

Plant

WINDOW

lavender

catnip

cayenne

lemon balm

climbing rose

orange tree

parsley

red clover

LOW TABLE

HANGING CHAIR WITH CUSHIONS

lovage

valerian

blue skullcap

N

St John's wort

German or Roman chamomile

sweet violet

peppermint

calendula

angelica

schisandra

TRELLIS

39

Propagating herbs

Whether your herb garden is in a soil bed or in pots, good propagation is key. Throughout the Guide, I've given basic advice on how to grow each herb. The following are the main methods of propagation you'll come across. (Many of the herbs in the Guide suggest germination in a greenhouse. If you don't have a greenhouse, a warm, sunny windowsill can work just as well.)

By seed: To propagate by seed sprinkle the seeds *in situ* in fine soil or (for precious or unfamiliar seeds) into a tray of seed compost to the depth of the seed, then sieve fine soil on top. Water in gently. When I suggest that you "surface-sow" the seeds, this means to scatter them on the soil's surface (light will trigger their germination) and sprinkle a little soil on top to anchor them.

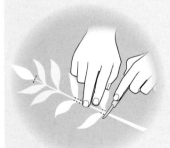

MAKING A CUTTING

Use this method to take cuttings of your plants. (The dotted lines denote cuts.)

1. Using a knife, slice the cutting just below a leaf junction, where clusters of growth cells will produce new roots.

2. Remove the leaves from the lower third of the cutting, slicing them with a knife.

3. Pinch out or snip off the growing tip (to encourage bushy growth), so you are left with only the parts shown in yellow.

For seeds sown in a tray, cover the tray with a glass lid to maintain moisture, and then with paper to prevent scorching. Check the tray daily and when seedlings appear, remove the paper and glass. When each seedling has six to 12 leaves, move the plants from the tray into individual small pots.

By plant division: Use this method mainly for perennials (see p.11). Dig up a mature plant and put two curved forks, back to back, in the centre of the plant's roots, to prise in half. Some plants are made up of a cluster of obvious little plants and you can divide these by separating them carefully by hand. In other species, you won't need to dig the plant at all, but should be able to slice away surface offshoots while it is in the ground. Whatever method you use, replant each piece in fresh soil, and water well until established.

By root, runner or rhizome sections: Take pieces of root, runner or rhizome that are 7½ to 20cm (3–8in) long, each with small hair roots and up to three buds. Plant the pieces just under the surface of fresh soil. Water regularly.

By cuttings: Cuttings (see also box, opposite) can be hardwood (woody pieces, taken in autumn to root over winter), softwood (new growth, taken in spring or summer), or flexible (half-ripened stems, taken in spring or summer). Most of the cuttings suggested in this book are softwood (flexible). Once you've taken a cutting, make a 15cm- (6in-) deep trench and half-fill with a sand-soil mix. Put the cuttings in the trench, fill in with soil and gently press to firm in around each cutting. Mist the leaves with water until roots develop.

Harvesting, drying and storing herbs

It's thoroughly satisfying to tend herbs, harvest them and put them to use. As a rule of thumb, pick your herbs on a warm, dry morning after the dew has evaporated. Choose herbs that you have positioned away from roadside pollution and pick only a maximum of one-third of the plant at a time. Harvest one type of herb at each session, to avoid any mix-ups. Wash the herbs only if absolutely necessary, and shake them dry.

For simplicity, in the Guide I've given harvesting information for only the parts of each plant that I use in the preparations. Check the harvesting and drying instructions below, before you go out to pick.

Leaves: For the best-quality leaves, pick just before flowering. Harvest large leaves individually, but, for ease, take whole stems of medium to small leaves. Dry your leaves gradually. In general, hang them upside-down inside, out of direct sunlight, in small bundles of between five and 10 stems. Drying will take about four days. Occasionally, you'll need to sun-dry the herbs – this quicker method preserves nutrients. To sun-dry, lay the leaves out individually, in the sunshine, on a muslin cloth. Once you have dried them (by either method), store the leaves whole, in clean dark-glass jars with airtight lids, to preserve their active ingredients (pick individual leaves off stems, if necessary). Label and date each jar; the herbs will normally last for six months kept out of sunlight. Condensation in the jar means that your leaves need more drying time.

Flowers: For larger flowers, such as calendula or rose, pick the flower heads individually at midday, when the flowers are fully opened. Remove any stalks and carefully lay each flower head on a muslin cloth that you've stretched over an empty frame (any frame will do). For small flowers that grow in clusters (such as elderflower) and stem flowers (such as lavender), pick whole stems and then hang them upside-down to dry (this may take up to three weeks). You can store whole, dried flowers, or you can pick off the dried petals. As with leaves, use a clean, airtight dark-glass jar, which you label and date, and keep out of direct sun. They'll usually last for three to six months.

Seeds: A plant's seeds are ripe when they are no longer green, and this is the best time to harvest them. Pick the whole stem, usually in late summer or autumn, and then hang the stem upside-down over a box to catch the seeds as they dry and fall off. The drying process usually takes about two weeks. Store for up to a year in lidded glass jars or paper envelopes, and label.

Roots: To harvest roots, dig them up as directed in the herb entries, clean them and cut them up into small pieces. Dry them by putting them in the stove on a low heat, turning them regularly until they break easily. Store the dried pieces for up to a year in a labelled and dated jar or paper bag.

Resins: A tree uses its sticky resin to "heal" wounds in its bark, protecting the inner trunk from microbes. To collect a resin, you need to "damage" the tree's bark to expose the sapwood (soft layers of wood beneath the bark), perhaps by scoring or scraping the trunk. Allow the resin to dry on the tree, then scrape it off. Store it in a paper bag. Resins will usually keep for several years.

Gardening for the spirit

When I think about a spiritual path, one of the most beautiful routes that comes to me is through nature – a trail as old as the planet itself. Standing in a sacred grove, early peoples felt the power of trees; when gathered around a protective night fire, they noticed that the fragrant smoke from the wood calmed their breathing and quietened their thoughts. Sacred trees – with their power and majesty – have touched us all, but the spiritual gifts of nature can be found in the smaller herbs, too.

This is why I believe it is so important to have a seat among your herbs (see pp.38–9). There are always more tasks to achieve than we have time for, so no matter what pressing deadlines you have, a seat encourages you to stop and enjoy the environment you've created, and to begin to make a deeper connection with nature.

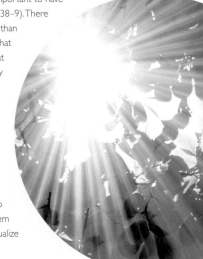

When you sit among your herbs, stroking them, tasting them or inhaling their fragrance, pause and allow your mind to expand into the core of just one herb. In your mind, travel down to its main roots and experience them establishing a firm foundation; visualize the fine hair roots searching for water and minerals; then feel the strength of the stem as it extends upward. Imagine being inside a new leaf opening in expectation of clean, fresh air, and of sunlight and raindrops; and, finally, notice how the herb grows to match an unseen blueprint. Soon, you'll become a more compassionate gardener, and your plant will return unexpected rewards.

Gifts from nature

When I have negative stress overloading my mind, I go and sit among my herbs. First comes an attempt to relax, to breathe deeply, unwinding into the space. For a while, this means simply observing the plant and insect activity around me – perhaps watching that persistent ladybird fall off the blade of grass again – until bit by bit my energy moves from stressed to neutral. By then, I am more open to the herbal atmosphere, and the vitality surrounding me starts to permeate my being, making me feel more positive. It's as if I've allowed my boundaries to become more porous. I come away feeling buoyant – with 100 new ideas – and the old stress, although not resolved, seems insignificant.

A spiritual journey with your herbs can be extended as much or as little as you wish. Playfully assume that each plant has something to teach you and aim to establish a rapport with the plant's essence. Begin with your favourite herb and connect with it through touch, scent or thought. Positive experiences can arise that have never been suggested to you, so you know your herb has a unique gift, just for you. I have one cheeky plant that sets me off telling jokes!

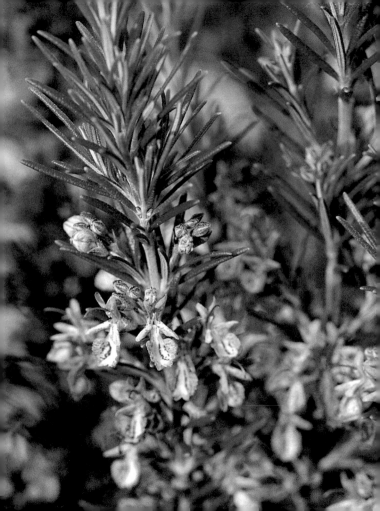

Part Two:
A Guide to Herbs

This section presents 105 herbs from around the world, including familiar garden plants, tropical trees, desert shrubs and an emperor's mushroom. The herbs are grouped into nine chapters, each focusing on a different aspect of the healing potential of herbs – from those that will energize your body in Chapter 1 to those that will lift and open up your spirit in Chapter 9. Discover the unique character of each herb through its origins, folklore and fascinating traditional uses. Learn how to grow and harvest the herbs and how to put each to practical use for physical, mental and spiritual well-being. The guide is an open treasure chest of herbs for you to explore, experiment with and enjoy.

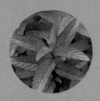 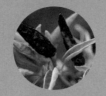 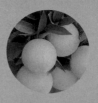

provide a stimulant for your heart and central nervous system.

However, the majority of my invigorators and stimulants come from plants that many of us know best as culinary spices – cayenne, cinnamon, nutmeg, clove and ginger. All these herbs revitalize the body by boosting circulation and warming the whole system. Most of them also increase levels of our digestive juices, to encourage the body to process food more efficiently and so increase levels of energy.

Of course, it's not just the body's physical systems that may be stimulated by the herbs in this chapter. Some of the plants featured have exotic histories as love potions to ignite passion, while others can stimulate mental energy or a more positive mood. Still others can induce a sense of the higher self, uplifting and exhilarating the spirit.

Cayenne *Capsicum frutescens*

"If you master only one herb in your life, make it cayenne pepper," teaches modern American herbalist Dr Schulze. This herb has the ability to "blow open" the circulation and deliver, sometimes within seconds, fresh blood, oxygen and nutrients to the whole body. Herbalists have saved heart-attack victims' lives with it. Cayenne's active ingredient, which stimulates the heart and circulation, is capsaicin (also a powerful digestive). It is present in both the *Capsicum frutescens* and *C. annuum* species of the plant. If you have a sensitive stomach, take only small amounts.

Plant type:
Evergreen perennial

Description: 1m (3ft) high by 1m (3ft) wide; bright red fruit

Native habitat: Tropical rainforest; C and S America

Parts of plant used:
Fruit, leaves

Growing and harvesting

- Requires well-drained soil in a hot, sunny position.
- Sow seeds in early spring in a greenhouse. Outside the Tropics, grow as an annual.
- Pick leaves any time, then dry; fruit when bright red. Or hang whole plant upside-down to dry crop.

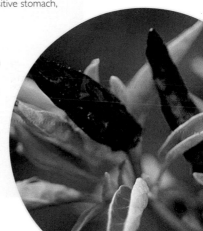

Lore and traditional uses
- Shamans included cayenne with their vision herbs to speed up contact with astral realms.
- Native Americans in Mexico use cayenne as an internal disinfectant against impure food.

Enhancing mind and spirit
- To keep alert during long drives, drink 60ml (2fl oz) grape, apple or tomato juice laced with a large pinch of cayenne powder.
- To heighten spiritual awareness, take 1 cup cayenne powder infusion (see first preparation, right) when required.

Caring for your body
- To fire the circulation and digestion, take up to ½ tsp cayenne power daily on food, or 1 size 00 capsule filled with cayenne powder (see p.21) three times daily with food.
- To treat chilblains, paint cayenne tincture (see second preparation, right) onto your toes.
- To ease cluster (recurring) headaches, heat cayenne leaves with a steam iron and apply the warmed leaves to your temples.

Core benefits

Stimulates circulation

Aids digestion

Painkilling

Preparations

Infusion: Stir ½–1 tsp cayenne powder into 1 cup just-boiled water. Sweeten with honey to taste.

Tincture: 60g (2oz) finely chopped fresh or dried cayenne pepper in 1 litre (2 pints) vodka-water mix. Standard method (p.20).

51

Cinnamon *Cinnamomum verum*

The young stems of this aromatic, evergreen tree, with their silky tassles of malodorous cream flowers, provide the popular spice cinnamon. The essential oil, which may be extracted from the tree's leaves, bark or roots, is added to food, toothpaste, chewing gum, incense and perfumes. Cinnamon powder has traditionally been used to stimulate digestion, ease indigestion and fight viral infections. Now this spice is the focus of exciting new research as a brain stimulant and blood-sugar regulator.

Plant type:
Evergreen tree

Description: 12m (40ft) tall by 10m (30ft) wide; small yellow-to-cream flowers

Native habitat: Tropical grassland; Sri Lanka

Parts of plant used:
Bark, essential oil (from leaves, bark or roots)

Growing and harvesting

- Tolerates many soil conditions in full or partial sun, but not frost. For best results, sow seeds in rich, moist soil in heat.
- When the plants are three years old, cut them back to just above ground to produce many young stems.
- Harvest finger-thick stems. Remove the inner cork and outer bark to leave inner bark, then dry and roll into quills.

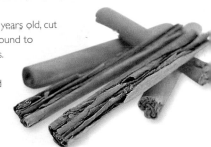

Lore and traditional uses

- The Roman emperor Nero burned a year's supply of cinnamon on his wife's funeral pyre.
- In African folk magic, cinnamon is used for purification, luck, love and to gain money.
- In Christian churches, aromatic candles were made using the fat from cinnamon seeds.

Enhancing mind and spirit

- To stimulate your zest for life, spray the space around you with a cinnamon room spray (see first preparation, right) as often as you wish.
- To aid memory, add ¼ tsp cinnamon powder to your favourite hot drink twice daily.

Caring for your body

- As an antibacterial for acne spots, mix 1 tsp honey with 1 tsp powdered cinnamon. Apply to the skin and leave overnight. Rinse off.
- To help stabilize blood sugar, add ¼–½ tsp cinnamon powder to your food twice daily.
- As an aphrodisiac, serve up a cinnamon-laced dessert, such as pumpkin pie, or cinnamon coffee (see second preparation, right).

Core benefits

Regulates blood sugar

Antimicrobial

Warming

Preparations

Room spray: In an atomizer, blend 3 drops cinnamon leaf essential oil with 25ml (1fl oz) water.

Cinnamon coffee: Whip ¼ cup whipping (heavy) cream with 1 tsp sugar, a pinch nutmeg and ⅛ tsp cinnamon powder. In a mug, stir 2 tsp chocolate syrup into ¾ cup hot coffee and top with the cinnamon-cream mix.

Lemon *Citrus limon*

As early as 700CE in the Middle East, lemon, with its perfumed flowers and aromatic leaves, was planted simply as an ornamental garden tree. Eventually the leaves came into use as flavouring and, in the 14th century, the Egyptians pressed the fruit to make what appears to be the first lemonade. We now know that refreshing lemon has an antibacterial and detoxifying juice that is highly therapeutic. The juiciest lemons have the smoothest skin and the smallest points at each end.

Plant type:
Evergreen tree

Description: 7m (23ft) tall by 6m (20ft) wide; white flowers; green leaves

Native habitat: Tropical rainforest; SE Asia

Parts of plant used:
Flowers, leaves, fruit, essential oil (from peel)

Growing and harvesting

- Trees require a well-drained, loamy soil in full sun. In cooler countries, pot-grow outdoors in summer and move indoors in winter.
- Sow seeds in a greenhouse and protect from frost for three or four winters. Or take cuttings of young, flexible stems between mid- and late summer; pot when rooted.
- Pick ripe fruit in autumn and use fresh, or freeze juice.

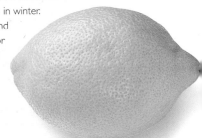

Lore and traditional uses

- In the 16th century, the Dutch East India Company gave lemon juice to its sailors every day to prevent scurvy.
- British colonialists in Singapore and Africa used lemon juice and leaves as substitutes for quinine in the treatment of malaria.

Enhancing mind and spirit

- To lift your spirits and stimulate your mind, place equal parts lemon juice and water in a spray bottle and use to refresh the air.

Caring for your body

- To give your system a master cleanse, fast for three days, but in that time drink 8 glasses of lemon detox drink (see first preparation, right) daily, as well as herbal teas and water.
- To soothe a sore throat, make a lemon throat syrup (see second preparation, right) and take it as often as you need until symptoms pass.
- To lighten age spots and tighten facial skin, dab the affected areas using a tissue soaked in lemon juice.

Core benefits

Refreshing

Cleansing

Antibacterial

Preparations

Detox drink: Mix 1 tbsp fresh lemon juice, 1 tbsp pure maple syrup and a few grains cayenne powder in a cup of pure water. Drink hot or cold.

Throat syrup: Skewer ½ a lemon and roast over a medium flame until the peel turns golden brown. Cool the lemon slightly, scoop out the pulp, mix with 1 tsp honey, then eat.

55

Orange *Citrus sinensis*

Next time you enjoy breakfast with a glass of refreshing orange juice or spread your toast with the tangy zest of orange marmalade, revel in all the good you are doing for your body. Brightly coloured fruits, such as oranges, burst with vitamins A and C, as well as minerals and antioxidants. This means that oranges help keep the eyes and skin healthy, maintain a strong heart, and boost the immune system, even protecting the body against some cancers.

Plant type:
Evergreen tree

Description: 9m (27ft) tall by 6m (18ft) wide; aromatic leaves and twigs

Native habitat: Tropical rainforest; SE Asia

Parts of plant used:
Flowers, leaves, fruit, essential oil (from peel), seed oil

Growing and harvesting

- Requires a moist, well-drained, loamy soil, and full sun.
- Sow seeds in a warm place and protect new plants from the cold for first few winters. Or propagate by taking cuttings of young, flexible stems in late summer Move roots carefully.
- Harvest leaves all year round, and pick ripe fruit in autumn.

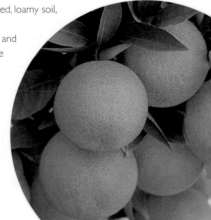

Lore and traditional uses

- In traditional Indian medicine, orange is used to purify the blood, allay thirst during fevers and treat catarrh, among other disorders.
- Orange peel's essential oil has long been used in flavourings, perfumery and cosmetics; the pressed seed oil is used in soaps.

Enhancing mind and spirit

- To lift your mood in the morning, place a few dried orange leaves in your clothes drawers to inhale their uplifting scent as you dress.
- To give a room a positive atmosphere, burn orange peel on an open fire.

Caring for your body

- To treat acne spots, peel an orange and rub the inner side of the rind over your face.
- To refresh the palate, steep 8 orange leaves in a cup of just-boiled water for 10 minutes, strain and then drink.
- To repel flies, ants, fleas and wasps, make a diluted citric peel oil insecticide (see preparation, right) and spray the room.

Core benefits

Stimulating

Uplifting

Insecticide

Preparation

Diluted citric peel oil insecticide: Using a paring knife, carefully peel the skin of an orange. Put the peel in a pan, cover with water and a lid and bring to a boil, then simmer for 10 minutes to release the insecticide oil. Strain the liquid into a small spray bottle.

Peppermint Mentha × piperita

Since ancient times, people all over the world have valued the refreshing, zingy taste of peppermint. Some claim that this plant is the world's most ancient medicine, as it has been found in archaeological sites more than 10,000 years old. Most varieties of mint are stimulant, digestive aids, but peppermint has additional antispasmodic and antimicrobial properties. Italian research in 2007 found that peppermint oil reduced irritable bowel symptoms in 75 percent of patients.

Plant type: Hardy creeping perennial

Description: 45cm (1½ft) high by 1m (3ft) wide; mid- to dark green leaves

Native habitat: All temperate; Eurasia, Africa

Parts of plant used: Leaves, essential oil (from leaves and small flowers)

Growing and harvesting

- Grows well in soil that is not too dry in sun or part shade.
- Propagate from a plant with good scent. In spring, take 15cm (6in) pieces of rhizome with a growing bud. Plant the pieces flat, 2.5cm (1in) deep in fresh soil.
- Harvest leaves and stems any time. Use fresh, or dry.

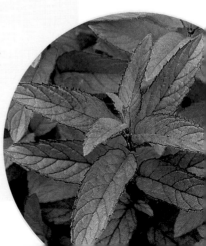

Lore and traditional uses

- In Greek myth, Minthe was a nymph loved by Hades, who transformed her into this scented herb to protect her from his jealous wife.
- In the Bible, the Pharisees are said to have collected tithes in mint, dill and cumin.

Enhancing mind and spirit

- To boost energy, add 4 cups peppermint leaf infusion (see first preparation, right) to a warm bath and soak for 20 minutes.
- To improve your memory and mental focus, spray the air around you with a refreshing peppermint-based room spray (see second preparation, right) as often as you like.

Caring for your body

- To reduce indigestion and flatulence, take 1 or 2 cups peppermint leaf infusion (see first preparation, right) after a meal.
- To curb the appetite, put 1 drop peppermint essential oil on a tissue; inhale before meals.
- To relax aching muscles, massage the areas with infused peppermint leaf oil (see p.23).

Core benefits

Stimulates digestion

Antimicrobial

Relieves muscle spasm

Preparations

Infusion: 1 tsp dried or 2 tsp fresh peppermint leaves in 1 cup just-boiled water. Standard method (p.20).

Room spray: In an atomizer blend 3 drops peppermint essential oil, 3 drops rosemary essential oil and 3 drops basil essential oil in 25ml (1fl oz) water.

Nutmeg *Myristica fragrans*

Nutmeg is one of the most highly prized spices in history – in 1667, the Dutch gave New Amsterdam (New York) to the British in exchange for the Moluccas, a rich source of nutmeg; and they threatened to execute anyone who stole a seed. This herb stimulates bloodflow and treats digestive disorders. Avoid taking more than ¾ tsp ground nutmeg daily.

Plant type:
Evergreen tree

Description: 20m (65ft) tall by 20m (65ft) wide; tiny yellow flowers

Native habitat: Tropical rainforest; Moluccas

Parts of plant used: Seeds, essential oil (from seeds)

Growing and harvesting
- Thrives in a hot, moist, climate, in well-drained soil with partial shade.
- Propagate both male and female trees from seed. Plant them singly in pots, then transplant when 22cm (9in) tall. One male tree will pollinate 10 to 12 females.
- Pick ripe fruit and then separate the nutmeg and mace to dry.

Lore and traditional uses
- One worldly 16th-century European monk told men

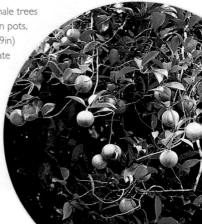

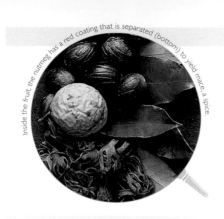

Inside the fruit, the nutmeg has a red coating that is separated (bottom) to yield mace, a spice.

Core benefits

Stimulates digestion

Aphrodisiac

Improves circulation

that to attract women they should anoint their genitalia with infused nutmeg oil.

Enhancing mind and spirit

- For a buoyant, mellow mood, add a pinch of nutmeg to your porridge in the morning.

Caring for your body

- To stimulate the heart and circulation, take 1 size 00 capsule filled with nutmeg powder (see p.21) twice daily.
- To aid digestion, take 1 cup nutmeg infusion (see first preparation, right) as required.
- To boost libido, drink a small glass of nutmeg liqueur (see second preparation, right) whenever necessary.

Preparations

Infusion: Grate a pinch nutmeg into 1 cup just-boiled water; sweeten to taste, then drink.

Nutmeg liqueur: Grate 1½ nutmegs into 600ml (1¼ pints) brandy or cognac. Steep for 3 weeks, then strain and bottle.

Guaraná *Paullinia cupana*

When I visited Manaus in the Amazon, my host kept a jar of powdered guaraná seed on the kitchen table, using it like a condiment in his food. For centuries, the Guaranis, an indigenous people of South America, have harvested the seeds of this plant to treat conditions as diverse as low libido, age-related memory loss, nervous tension, and obesity. The active compounds in the seed include theophyline, which stimulates the heart and central nervous system, and caffeine. Avoid guaraná if you suffer from caffeine sensitivity, are taking anticoagulant medications, or are pregnant or breastfeeding.

Growing and harvesting

- Requires a hot, moist environment in acidic soil and full sun.
- Sow seeds immediately (they lose viability within three days) in a warm place; or if you are propagating from cuttings, keep them in a mist chamber.
- Harvest seeds when fruit is overripe, then roast, peel and grind them. Store in sealed glass jars as a powder.

Plant type: Climbing woody vine

Description: Up to 12m (40ft) long; tiny white flower clusters; red fruits

Native habitat: Tropical rainforest; Brazilian Amazon

Parts of plant used: Seeds, essential oil (from seed)

Preparations

Infusion: 1 tsp soluble guaraná powder in 1 cup just-boiled water. Standard method (p.20).

Tincture: 200g (7oz) powdered guaraná seed in 1 litre (2 pints) water. Standard method (p.20).

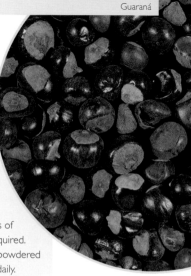

Lore and traditional uses

- The Guarani tribe use this herb to restore their vigour and energy.
- Guaraná is the main ingredient in Brazil's "national beverage" – guaraná soda.

Enhancing mind and spirit

- To stimulate energy, stir 1 tsp powdered guaraná seed into a glass of your favourite juice and drink as required.
- To enhance memory, take 2–3 tsp powdered guaraná seed on food or in drinks daily.

Caring for your body

- To detoxify the blood, take 1 cup guaraná powder infusion or ½ tsp tincture in a little water (see preparations, left) or 1 size 00 capsule filled with powdered guaraná seed (see p.21) up to three times daily.
- To help reduce cellulite, stir ½ tsp guaraná tincture (see second preparation, left) into your usual body lotions and apply daily.

Core benefits
Stimulates energy
Enhances memory
Weight loss

Clove *Syzygium aromaticum*

In China, the clove – the sun-dried, unopened flower bud of the dense, evergreen clove tree – is called *dingxiang* or "tiny thing that makes a good smell". Its fiery pungency is used in perfumery, in Traditional Chinese Medicine as a "hot" remedy, and as a catalyst to activate other therapeutic herbs. As a food flavouring, clove provides a stimulating digestive that reduces nausea, stomach pains and intestinal gas, and a strong antimicrobial that both protects the body and preserves food.

Plant type:
Evergreen tree

Description: 20m (65ft) tall by 10m (3ft) wide; small, cream flower heads

Native habitat: Tropical rainforest; Moluccas

Parts of plant used: Flowers, essential oil (from clove bud)

Growing and harvesting

- Requires well-drained, rich, moist soil in humidity and warm full or partial sun.
- Dig soil with ample compost and rotted manure before planting seeds or cuttings. Keep well watered during dry periods.
- After the eighth year, pick unopened flower buds twice a year and sun-dry.

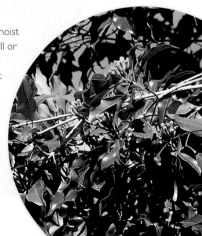

Lore and traditional uses

- Ayurvedic healers use clove as an aphrodisiac – a use supported by scientific research.
- Clove is traditionally used to numb toothache, which has led to new clove-based anesthetics.

Enhancing mind and spirit

- To stimulate mental energy, add a pinch of clove powder to hot tea, coffee or milk.
- To give a warming atmosphere to your workspace in winter, put ½ cup pure water in a spray bottle and add 2 drops clove essential oil. Spray the air as often as you like.
- To provide a welcoming aroma for visitors to your home, hang a clove pomander (see first preparation, right) in your hallway.

Caring for your body

- To stimulate digestion and reduce nausea and flatulence, add a pinch of clove powder to your favourite digestive herbal tea.
- To fight diarrhea and intestinal parasites, take 1 cup clove infusion (see second preparation, right) up to three times daily, as necessary.

Core benefits

Stimulates digestion

Anesthetic

Antimicrobial

Preparations

Pomander: Stick 60–100 cloves into the skin of a ripe orange, in an attractive pattern. Leave enough space around the middle of the orange to tie a ribbon by which to hang your pomander.

Infusion: 1 tsp powdered clove in 1 cup just-boiled water. Standard method (p.20).

Alecost *Tanacetum balsamita*

Alecost leaves have a clean, invigorating, spearmint-like scent, and before the use of hops were used to clarify, preserve and flavour ale, giving the herb the first part of its name. The "cost" part derives from the Greek *kostos*, meaning a spicy, Oriental herb. Alecost's other common names are costmary, meaning Mary's (women's) spicy herb in reference to its use to ease childbirth; and bible leaf, because Puritans kept alecost leaves inside their Bibles so the aroma would ward off hunger during sermons.

Plant type:
Hardy perennial

Description: 1m (3ft) high by 1m (3ft) wide; white, daisy-like flowers

Native habitat: Cool temperate; Europe, Asia

Parts of plant used: Leaves

Growing and harvesting

- Grows easily in rich, well-drained soil in full sun or part shade.
- Fails to seed in cooler climates, but where available, sow seeds in spring. In other areas, propagate by dividing roots in spring or autumn.
- Pick leaves while young, from spring to early autumn. Use fresh, or dry for later use.

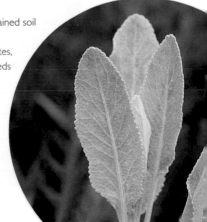

Lore and traditional uses

- During medieval times, alecost leaves were strewn on the floor and added to pot pourri to refresh the air and repel insects.

Enhancing mind and spirit

- To stimulate and refresh your spirit, enjoy a cup of alecost leaf infusion (see first preparation, right) whenever you wish.
- For a fragrant surprise, place dried alecost leaves in a coat-hanger bag in your closet or in a sofa sack (see second preparation, right), so you inhale the uplifting scent when you are dressing or relaxing, and least expect it.

Caring for your body

- To ease a stuffy nose, try an alecost steam inhalation, using a handful of fresh alecost leaves in a bowl of boiling water (see p.22).
- To relieve a bee sting, apply a bruised alecost leaf to the affected area.
- To ease the pain of childbirth, take 1 cup alecost leaf infusion (see first preparation, right), three times daily during a long labour.

Core benefits

Refreshing

Enhances body systems

Insecticide

Preparations

Infusion: 1 tsp dried or 3 tsp fresh alecost leaves in 1 cup just-boiled water. Standard method (p.20).

Sofa sack: Make 2 small gauze pillows and stuff each with dried alecost leaves; sew closed. Sew the pillows onto opposite ends of two 90cm (3ft) long ribbons, which you then hang over the back of the sofa.

Ginger *Zingiber officinale*

In Ayurvedic medicine, ginger is called the "universal medicine", because it has the ability to heal such a wide range of ailments. The plant's spicy rhizome (underground stem) stimulates the circulation to create warmth and an overall feeling of well-being. It also aids every part of the digestive process, reduces joint inflammation and treats nausea.

Growing and harvesting

- Needs fertile soil, moisture and a temperature of at least 28°C (82°F) all year.
- In spring, plant fresh, firm rhizome pieces, each with two growing buds, in pots or in the ground, 2.5cm (1in) deep, in filtered light.
- Once plump, unearth rhizome in late autumn. Use fresh, or sun-dry.

Lore and traditional uses

- In China, for more than 3,000 years, ginger has been considered a *yang* tonic to boost energy and warm colds and chills.

Plant type:
Creeping perennial

Description: 1m (3ft) high; dense spikes of fragrant white flowers

Native habitat: Tropical rainforest; SE Asia, Jamaica

Parts of plant used:
Rhizome, essential oil (from rhizome)

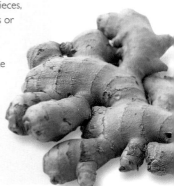

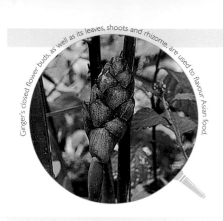

Ginger's closed flower buds, as well as its leaves, shoots and rhizome, are used to flavour Asian food.

Core benefits

Stimulates digestion

Boosts circulation

Reduces nausea

Enhancing mind and spirit

- To feel energized about life, in an atomizer, blend 3 drops each ginger, peppermint and orange essential oils with 25ml (1fl oz) water and spray around your space as required.

Caring for your body

- To relieve acid reflux, or intestinal gas or cramps, take 1 cup ginger infusion (see first preparation, right) three times daily.
- To warm up feet, rub them with 3 drops each ginger, black pepper and cinnamon essential oils in 4 tsp sweet almond oil twice daily.
- For travel sickness, take 1 tsp ginger tincture (see second preparation, right) in a little water or juice up to three times daily.

Preparations

Infusion: Steep 1 tsp dried ginger powder or 2.5cm (1in) grated fresh ginger root in 1 cup just-boiled water for 5 minutes. Strain. Add lemon to taste.

Tincture: 200g (7oz) dried ginger powder or 400g (14oz) grated fresh ginger root in 1 litre (2 pints) vodka-water mix. Standard method (p.20).

CHAPTER 2

Brain Tonics

When it's time to engage in mental activity, two types of herb will particularly help improve your concentration: clean, crisp aromatics that clear and focus the mind, marshall the brain and refresh the spirit, and herbs that work at a cellular level in the brain to increase oxygen uptake and in turn promote mental clarity.

The first group comprises herbs that have clean, green scents with a hint of sharpness (no floral fragrances here)

– try rosemary, basil, angelica or bay. Their scents will focus your mind and help you concentrate. If your job involves long hours of concentration – say at a computer or a checkout counter – try putting several fresh sprigs in a vase at your work station. Every time you need a mental refresher, take a deep breath of one the sprigs, or pinch its leaves between your fingers and then inhale the aroma it releases. See

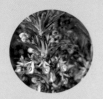
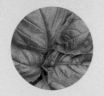
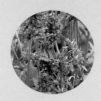

how the scent instantly revives
and re-energizes you.

The second group – which
includes the herbs brahmi, gotu
kola and ginkgo – are perhaps
even more remarkable. Their
proven ability to improve
brain-cell function not only
makes them great for toning
your memory and powers of
recall – say for an exam (see
box, p.27) or to make you
more efficient at your job
– but research shows they
also have exciting potential
to rejuvenate the brain. These
herbs appear to reduce
age-related memory loss,
and some, such as gingko and
brahmi, also provide nerve
tonics that may help inhibit
diseases of the central nervous
system, such as Alzheimer's
or Parkinson's disease.

Whether you are looking
to improve concentration or
to keep your mind youthful,
the herbs in this chapter will
provide you with an arsenal
of possibilities.

Angelica *Angelica archangelica*

This noble herb has a lush, tropical appearance and blooms with large spheres of flowers in midsummer. In the Northern hemisphere, this coincides with the early Christian feast day of the Archangel Michael, from which the herb derives its name. Angelica's reputation as a mind tonic comes mainly from its large leaves, which are sharp-scented and refreshing to smell. Research has found that the root contains 12 anti-inflammatory, 10 muscle-relaxant and five pain-relieving constituents. Avoid angelica if you are pregnant.

Plant type: Three-year hardy biennial

Description: 2m (6ft) high by 1m (3ft) wide; large leaves; green-white flowers

Native habitat: Cool temperate; N and E Europe

Parts of plant used: Roots, leaves, seeds, thin stems

Growing and harvesting

- Plant fresh seeds in late summer in deep, moist soil in light shade.
- Harvest leaves before the plant flowers to use fresh, or dry; and gather the seeds when ripe in early autumn, then dry.
- Dig up root in autumn of the plant's first year, then leave to dry before using.

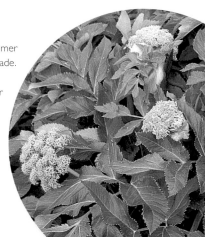

Lore and traditional uses

- Medieval choir wardens fumigated choir gowns with smoke from smouldering angelica.
- Angelica's tangy seeds and roots are traditionally used to flavour vermouth and gin.

Enhancing mind and spirit

- To refresh the brain during a monotonous task, such as a long car journey, inhale the scent of crushed, fresh angelica leaves.
- For a spiritual tonic to harmonize the *chakras* or meridians, put 4–7 drops angelica flower essence (see pp.34–5) under your tongue.

Caring for your body

- For a liver detox, drink ½ cup angelica decoction (see first preparation, right) three times daily for two to three weeks.
- To ease painful joints, apply a compress made with double-strength angelica decoction (see first preparation, right), as required.
- To ease the muscles, soak in a bath laced with 500ml (1 pint) double-strength angelica leaf infusion (see second preparation, right).

Core benefits

Protective

Balancing

Anti-inflammatory

Preparations

Decoction: 30g (1oz) dried or 60g (2oz) fresh angelica root in 750ml (1½ pints) water. Standard method (p.20). (For double strength, use 60g/2oz dried or 120g/4oz fresh in 750ml/1½ pints water.)

Double-strength infusion: 2 tsp dried or 4 tsp fresh leaves in 1 cup just-boiled water. Standard method (p.20).

Brahmi *Bacopa monnieri*

In Ayurvedic medicine, brahmi (also known as bacopa) has been used for more than 3,000 years as a *medhya* herb, one taken specifically for the mind. It increases circulation to the brain and supplies the brain with a protein (Bacoside B) known to nourish nerve cells. Students in India use brahmi to improve their memory and mental clarity. Brahmi grows beautifully in hanging baskets, where its stems will cascade over the sides for easy picking.

Growing and harvesting

- Propagate brahmi by seed, cuttings or root division in moist soil in pots. As brahmi is a shallow-rooting bog plant, place the pots in a tray of water.
- Outside the Tropics, grow brahmi as an annual, and feed the plant with seaweed fertilizer in the growing season.
- Harvest sprigs of leaves any time.

Lore and traditional uses

- In India, small amounts of brahmi infusion are given to infants to promote mental

Plant type:
Perennial

Description: 10cm (4in) high; ground cover; fleshy leaves; white flowers

Native habitat: Tropical rainforest; India

Parts of plant used: Leaves

Preparations

Infusion: Six 9cm (3½in) brahmi sprigs in 1 cup just-boiled water. Standard method (p.20).

Tincture: 75g (2½oz) dried, powdered brahmi leaves in 1 litre (2 pints) vodka-water mix. Standard method (p.20).

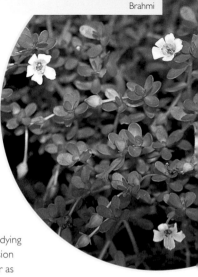

development. The tea is given daily to the elderly to rejuvenate the brain.

- Brahmi's ability to promote focus and a sense of calm have made it a popular traditional aid to meditation.

Enhancing mind and spirit

- To balance the two sides of the brain during meditation, or to enhance mental capacity while studying for exams, take 1 cup brahmi infusion (see first preparation, left) daily, for as long as necessary.

Caring for your body

- To keep the brain cells young, beginning well before old age, take 1 cup brahmi infusion (see first preparation, left), or take 1 tsp brahmi tincture (see second preparation, left) in water daily, as required.
- To boost the circulation, add fresh brahmi leaves to salads regularly.

Core benefits

Enhances memory

Boosts circulation

Aids immunity

Gotu kola *Centella asiatica*

Known in India as "food for the brain", this remarkable herb improves reflexes, reduces stress and depression and promotes mental clarity. It can also increase energy – the 10th-century Sri Lankan king, Aruna, claimed that it gave him the stamina to satisfy his entire 50-woman harem. The plant loves rocky places and is often found growing on old stone walls. As well as taking gotu kola as an infusion or decoction, you can add a small number of the raw leaves to salads, or cook them in curries.

Plant type:
Perennial

Description: 40cm (16in) high by 40cm (16in) wide; small leaves

Native habitat: Tropical grassland; India, SE Asia

Parts of plant used: Leaves, stems

Growing and harvesting

- Prefers moist soil in sun or partial shade.
- Plant seeds in seed compost in a greenhouse, then re-pot individually when each young plant has two pairs of leaves. Move outdoors in late spring or early summer.
- Harvest leaves or stems any time.

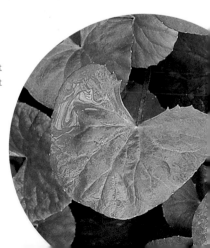

Lore and traditional uses

- Hindus often use gotu kola as a meditation aid to increase their understanding of Brahman, the supreme reality.
- Gotu kola is part of the Taoist Elixir taken by the Tai Chi master Li Ching-Yun, who died in 1933, chronicled to be 256 years old.

Enhancing mind and spirit

- To ease stress and relieve exhaustion, take 2–4 tsp gotu kola tincture (see first preparation, right) in a little water three times daily.
- For mental clarity, take 3 cups gotu kola leaf infusion (see second preparation, right) daily.

Caring for your body

- To fight premature aging, and to benefit from this herb's superb antioxidant properties, take 3 cups gotu kola leaf infusion (see second preparation, right) daily.
- To reduce wound scarring, apply a few drops gotu kola leaf-and-stem infused oil (see p.23) to the affected skin two or three times daily while the wound is still inflamed.

Core benefits

Aids mental function

Rejuvenates brain cells

Heals wounds

Preparations

Tincture: 200g (7oz) dried or 400g (14oz) fresh gotu kola leaves in 1 litre (2 pints) vodka-water mix. Standard method (p.20).

Infusion: 1 tsp dried or 2 tsp fresh gotu kola leaves in 1 cup just-boiled water. Standard method (p.20).

Ginkgo *Ginkgo biloba*

Having grown on Earth for more than 300 million years, ginkgo is our most ancient tree species. Each tree can live for up to 1,000 years. Ginkgo's therapeutic leaves protect against a broad range of age-related illnesses, including cataracts, strokes and heart disease. Many studies verify ginkgo's ability to improve brain function and to slow memory loss: it increases the oxygen uptake of all the body's cells, including the brain's. Avoid ginkgo if you are taking blood-thinning medication.

Plant type: Hardy deciduous tree

Description: 30m (100ft) tall by 20m (65ft) wide; fan-shaped, small leaves

Native habitat: Cool temperate; E China

Parts of plant used: Leaves

Growing and harvesting

- Prefers moist, deep, well-drained sandy soil in full sun to part shade, with wind shelter.
- Grow the tree from seed (found within the yellow fruits) in a warm place for the first year.
- Harvest leaves any time in spring, summer or early autumn, before they turn yellow.

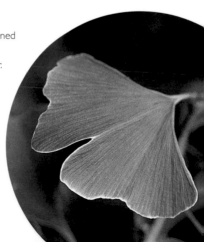

Lore and traditional uses

- In China around 3,000BCE, ginkgo was noted for its ability to increase sexual energy.
- In China, Korea and Japan, ginkgo is a venerated tree, grown in temple gardens.

Enhancing mind and spirit

- For a speedy brain boost, infuse 1 tsp ginkgo-based blend (see first preparation, right) in 1 cup just-boiled water. Drink up to 3 cups of this blend daily.
- To enhance your memory of dreams, take 1 cup half-strength ginkgo leaf infusion (see second preparation, right) before bedtime.

Caring for your body

- To increase libido in both men and women, take 1–3 cups ginkgo leaf infusion (see second preparation, right) or one size 00 capsule filled with powdered ginkgo leaf (see p.21) daily.
- To inhibit allergic responses, such as hay fever, take one size 00 capsule filled with powdered ginkgo leaf (see p.21) daily, as required.

Core benefits

Improves memory

Increases circulation

Enhances libido

Preparations

Ginkgo-based blend: Mix together 4½ tsp each dried ginkgo powder and gotu kola powder and 1 tsp cayenne powder. Store in an airtight container.

Infusion: 1 tsp dried or 3 tsp fresh ginkgo leaves in 1 cup just-boiled water. Standard method (p.20). (For half-strength, use ½ tsp dried or 1½ tsp fresh leaves.)

Bay *Laurus nobilis*

In ancient Greece, the Delphi priestess inhaled the mildly narcotic aroma of bay when she received the prophecies of the god Apollo – establishing bay as an important herb for all matters relating to the mind and higher learning. In modern times, we know that bay contains compounds called parthenolides, which help relieve migraines. The leaves also contain antispasmodic properties that can ease stomach pain and aid digestion, as well as relieve muscular pain.

Growing and harvesting

- Prefers a well-drained, light soil in sun or partial shade.
- In autumn, take mature 12.5–15cm (5–6in) side shoots cut through the swelling where shoot joins stem. Plant under cover (such as in a net tunnel) for 18 months, then plant out.
- Harvest leaves any time. Use dry.

Lore and traditional uses

- The ancient Greeks used wreaths of bay to honour scholars and Olympic athletes.

Plant type: Hardy evergreen tree

Description: 12m (36ft) tall by 8m (25ft) wide; small, cream flowers; blue berries

Native habitat: Warm temperate; Mediterranean

Parts of plant used: Leaves

Preparations

Cushion: Take a gauze rectangle (30cm/12in long by 21cm/8in wide). Fold it over and sew up two sides, leaving the other side open. Fill with dried bay leaves, then sew up the opening.

Decoction: Simmer 2 cupfuls dried bay leaves in 2 litres (4 pints) water for 15 minutes. Strain (you'll have about 1 litre/2 pints liquid).

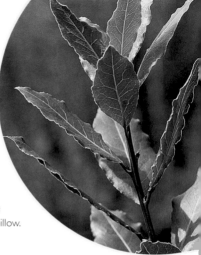

- The Roman Emperor Tiberius clutched a laurel wreath during thunderstorms to protect himself against lightning.

Enhancing mind and spirit

- To increase your psychic ability, inhale the smoke of smouldering bay leaves.
- To encourage prophetic dreams, sleep with a small bay cushion (see first preparation, left) under your pillow.

Caring for your body

- To halt a migraine, steam-iron several bay leaves and rest with the warmed leaves on your forehead for around 45 minutes.
- To aid digestion, add a few bay leaves to bouquet garni, marinades, soups and stews. Remove them before eating.
- To relieve aching limbs and joints, pour 1 litre (2 pints) bay decoction (see second preparation, left) into a warm bath and soak in it for 20 minutes.

Core benefits

Protective

Relieves pain

Aids digestion

Basil *Ocimum basilicum*

Basil's spicy scent is particularly intense in the herb's essential oil, which is used to revive a fainting spell, improve concentration and stimulate a sense of smell that has been dulled by viral infection. This herb provides many nutrients, including vitamins A and C and antioxidants, which all help improve eyesight and boost the health of the skin, hair and heart. Avoid using basil essential oil directly on your skin and during pregnancy.

Plant type:
Tender annual

Description: 45cm (1½ft) high by 30cm (1ft) wide; green or purple leaves

Native habitat: Tropical rainforest; Asia

Parts of plant used: Leaves, flowers, essential oil (from leaves)

Growing and harvesting
- Prefers a light, well-drained soil in sun.
- Sow seeds thinly in a greenhouse to avoid cold and damp.
- Water the soil, rather than the leaves, around midday.
- Harvest leaves all summer.

Lore and traditional uses
- In Mexico, basil is put in the pockets of a lover with a roving eye, to refocus his or her affections.

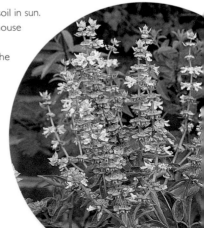

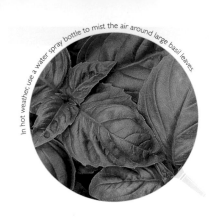

In hot weather, use a water spray bottle to mist the air around large basil leaves.

Core benefits

Refreshing

Focusing

Antioxidant

Enhancing mind and spirit

- To refresh the mind, put 1 drop basil essential oil on a tissue and inhale.
- To enhance memory and concentration, soak 10 fresh basil leaves in 1 cup cold water overnight. In the morning, strain and drink.

Caring for your body

- To reduce the itching of an insect bite, rub a fresh basil leaf onto the area, as required.
- To clear the head during a head cold, use a basil steam inhalation (see first preparation, right) until symptoms are relieved.
- To improve libido, drink a sherry glassful of basil tonic wine (see second preparation, right), as required.

Preparations

Inhalation: 2 tbsp dried or a handful fresh basil leaves in 5 litres (3 pints) water. Standard method (p.22).

Tonic wine: 100g (3½oz) dried or 200g (7oz) fresh basil leaves in 1 litre (2 pints) red wine. Standard method (p.22).

Black pepper *Piper nigrum*

One of the world's oldest traded spices, black pepper has a sharp, invigorating taste and a scent that promotes mental clarity. Although it is known primarily as a flavouring, in Ayurvedic medicine black pepper has been used for 4,000 years to warm the body and restore vitality. The 5th-century *Book of Medicines* from Syria prescribes pepper for 20 ailments, including constipation, diarrhea, earache and toothache.

Plant type:
Perennial vine

Description: Up to 6m (18ft) long; heart-shaped leaves

Native habitat: Tropical grassland; S India, Sri Lanka

Parts of plant used: Berries, essential oil (from crushed black peppercorns)

Growing and harvesting

- Grows best in rich, alluvial soils in bright, filtered light.
- Sow seeds in a greenhouse in loam compost with added sand. Maintain high humidity during the spring or summer growing season and feed monthly. Water sparingly during winter.
- Peppercorns may take several years to appear. To make black pepper, harvest green peppercorns as they appear, then dry.

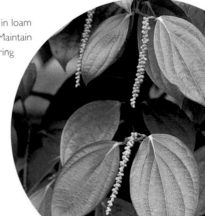

Lore and traditional uses

- In medieval Europe, peppercorns were so valued that they were accepted as payment for dowries, taxes and rents.
- Homeopaths traditionally use black pepper to aid concentration and banish apprehension.

Enhancing mind and spirit

- To enhance mental clarity, put 3 drops black pepper essential oil on a tissue and periodically inhale.

Caring for your body

- To energize aching, stiff muscles, apply a black-pepper-based massage oil (see first preparation, right) to the affected areas using long, firm strokes.
- To stimulate the body with a detoxifying body wash, make a black pepper soap (see second preparation, right) and use it in your morning shower every day.
- To get your gastric juices going and aid digestion, sprinkle your food liberally with freshly ground black pepper.

Core benefits

Stimulating

Energizing

Warming

Preparations

Massage oil: Blend 4 drops black pepper, 3 drops rosemary and 3 drops lavender essential oils in 4 tsp sweet almond oil.

Soap: Add 10 drops each black pepper and lavender essential oils to a bottle of 200ml (6½fl oz) unscented liquid soap; stir with a wooden chopstick. Soap will last indefinitely.

Rosemary *Rosmarinus officinalis*

Rosemary stimulates the brain's nervous system and boosts blood circulation. The herb contains antioxidants that aid memory and protect the body against free radicals, which damage the body's cells. One of rosemary's antioxidants is carnosic acid, which has a unique, particularly potent method of protection. Avoid rosemary essential oil during pregnancy.

Plant type: Hardy evergreen shrub

Description: 1.5m (5ft) high by 1.5m (5ft) wide; pale blue flowers

Native habitat: Warm temperate; Mediterranean

Parts of plant used: Leaves, stems, flowers, essential oil (from leaves)

Growing and harvesting
• Prefers light soil and full sun.
• Grow from 15cm (6in) cuttings in spring.
• Harvest leaves any time. Use fresh, or dry.

Lore and traditional uses
• In Europe, rosemary was once woven into wedding wreaths to represent fidelity.

Enhancing mind and spirit
• To aid creativity and ease the emotions, put 2 drops rosemary flower essence

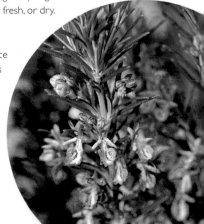

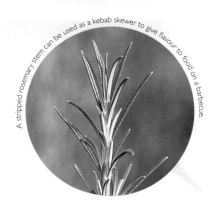

A stripped rosemary stem can be used as a kebab skewer to give flavour to food on a barbecue.

(see pp.34–5) in a glass of water and sip frequently throughout the day.

- To ease mental fatigue, make 1 cup rosemary leaf infusion (see first preparation, right), inhale the steam, and then drink.

Caring for your body

- To ease sore muscles, add 3 drops rosemary essential oil to a bath; soak for 20 minutes.
- For dandruff, rinse your hair with rosemary leaf infusion (see first preparation, right).

Special tip

Use a strong rosemary decoction (see second preparation, right) as a household antiseptic cleaner for kitchens and bathrooms.

Core benefits

Uplifting

Aids memory

Stimulates circulation

Preparations

Infusion: 1 tsp dried or 2 tsp fresh rosemary leaves in 1 cup just-boiled water. Standard method (p.20).

Strong decoction: 60g (2oz) dried or 120g (4oz) fresh rosemary leaves in 750ml (1½ pints) water. Standard method (p.20).

Wood betony *Stachys officinalis*

European wood betony (as opposed to the North American *Pedicularis canadensis*, also known as wood betony) is a cerebral tonic that tones and strengthens the nervous system. It has been employed medicinally for centuries – John Gerard's *Great Herbal* of 1597 gives it more than 29 uses. Today, herbalists use this herb to treat headaches and improve poor memory and to alleviate nervous tension.

Growing and harvesting
- Prefers to grow in a light, moist soil in full sun or part shade.
- Sow seeds in spring. Divide the grown plant at any time of year, except during frost.
- Collect aerial parts during flowering.

Lore and traditional uses
- The Druids used wood betony to expel evil, banish nightmares and overcome despair.
- The physician attending the Roman emperor Caesar Augustus noted 47 ailments that are cured by wood betony, including headaches.

Plant type:
Hardy perennial

Description: 60cm (2ft) high by 45cm (1½ft) wide; red or purple flowers

Native habitat: Cool temperate; Europe

Parts of plant used: Dried aerial parts

Preparations

Tonic wine: 100g (3½oz) wood betony's dried aerial parts in 1 litre (2 pints) red wine. Standard method (p.22).

Double-strength infusion: 2 tsp wood betony's dried aerial parts in 1 cup just-boiled water. Standard method (p.20).

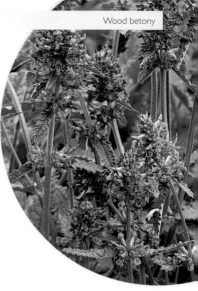

Enhancing mind and spirit

- To strengthen the crown and sacral *chakras* (see p.17) and fortify resolve during celibacy, put 2 drops wood betony flower essence (see pp.34–5) in a glass of water and sip throughout the day.
- To reduce nightmares, fill a small cloth pillow with dried wood betony and place this under your ordinary pillow as you sleep.

Caring for your body

- To ease nervous headaches, drink a sherry glassful of wood betony tonic wine (see first preparation, left) once a day before a meal, until your symptoms have passed.
- To relieve a sore throat, gargle with ½ cup double-strength wood betony infusion (see second preparation, left) three times daily.
- To provoke strong sneezing to relieve sinus headaches and treat nasal congestion, inhale a pinch of dried wood betony as a herbal snuff.

Core benefits

Relieves headaches

Nerve tonic

Protective

CHAPTER 3

Immune Enhancers

The world around us constantly bombards our bodies with bacteria, viruses, fungi and parasites. A strong immune system is our vital defence against all these potential invaders.

Good immunity must accomplish two things. First, it must recognize harmful foreign invaders; and, second, it must quickly stop them from attacking our body's cells.

Improving your mood (a buoyant attitude helps repel illness), your diet and your lifestyle helps keep you firmly on the path to good health. Not only can herbs provide high levels of vitamins and minerals to enhance nutrition, and mood-altering fragrances to lift your spirits, but crucially, many herbs also directly help the immune system launch and sustain its attack on invaders.

The human body has evolved an army of different types of fighter cells to keep it healthy, and every herb in

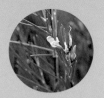 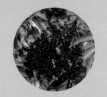 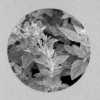

this chapter works uniquely to boost one or more of them.

For example, garlic increases the numbers of killer cells in the body (these help reject tumour- and virus-infected cells). Elderberry triggers the body's chemical messengers that stop viruses replicating. Garlic and astragalus mobilize "search-and-destroy" cells, called macrophages, which roam through the body, ingesting harmful invaders, fragmenting them and spitting them out so they can be whisked away by helper T-cells. These T-cells are themselves boosted by the wonderful immunity herb, echinacea.

Meanwhile, pau d'arco brings equilibrium to the immune system when treatments such as chemotherapy cause it to become imbalanced.

Increasingly, scientific research validates the idea that herbs can boost immunity. This chapter is your very own clinic for longlasting good health.

Garlic *Allium sativum*

Nature's own bodyguard, garlic is a superb antimicrobial. Its medicinal pedigree starts with Sumerian clay tablets dating from 2600BCE, while Egyptian papyri from 1500BCE list 22 therapeutic recipes that use garlic, including remedies to improve stamina. Studies in Russia and Japan have found that, in the body, garlic binds to heavy metals, including lead, mercury and cadmium, aiding their elimination.

Plant type:
Hardy perennial bulb

Description: 45cm (1½ft) high by 15cm (6in) wide; small bulbs at stem ends

Native habitat: Cool temperate; central Asia

Part of plant used: Bulb

Growing and harvesting
- Prefers moist, well-drained soil and sun.
- Plant individual garlic cloves 4cm (1½in) deep in late autumn.
- Once grown, stop watering the plant to allow it to dry out. Dig up the bulb in early summer.
- Hang bulb to dry fully, or preserve in oil or vinegar.

Lore and traditional uses
- Garlic has a reputation as a protector against evil, especially vampires.

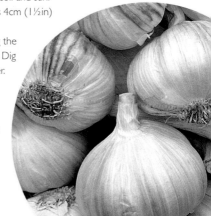

- European folklore suggested that people put garlic in a small bag and tie the bag around a child's neck to protect against a cold, or around the tummy to protect against worms.
- During World War I, British army doctors squeezed raw garlic juice directly onto wounds to successfully control infections.

Enhancing mind and spirit

- To strengthen objectivity, releasing fear, paranoia and anger, put 2 drops garlic flower essence (see pp.34–5) in a glass of water and sip frequently throughout the day.

Caring for your body

- To halt a cold or the flu, on the night of the first signs of illness sleep with a garlic bandage (see first preparation, right) wrapped around each foot.
- To help lower cholesterol levels or blood pressure, take 1 size 00 capsule filled with garlic powder (see p.21) or 1 tsp garlic tincture (see second preparation, right) in a little water twice daily, as necessary.

Core benefits

Antibiotic

Lowers cholesterol

Detoxifying

Preparations

Bandage: Crush a clove of garlic and place it in the centre of a length of bandage. Secure the bandage around your foot so the garlic is held in place against the skin on your sole. Repeat for the other foot.

Tincture: 200g (7oz) peeled garlic cloves in 1 litre (2 pints) vodka-water mix. Standard method (p.20).

Rooibos *Aspalathus linearis*

Native to the Western Cape of South Africa, rooibos (pronounced roy-boss and meaning "red bush") is a gorse-like shrub with leaves that offer a pleasant-tasting, caffeine-free tea. Tests show that this tea restricts damage to the body's DNA (the first stage of cancer) and encourages the body to produce two enzymes that are potent detoxifiers. Early studies show that rooibos also aids antibody production, helping prevent allergies and viral infections.

Plant type: Shrub; perennial legume

Description: 1.5m (5ft) high by 1m (3ft) wide; tiny, yellow, pea-like flowers

Native habitat: Tropical grassland; South Africa

Parts of plant used: Leaves, small stems

Growing and harvesting

- Needs a well-drained, acidic, sandy soil in full sun. Grows best in a hot, dryish climate at altitudes above 150m (500ft).

- In late spring, soak seeds for 12 hours in warm water, then sow in a greenhouse just below the surface of the soil.

- Pinch out tips of the plant to encourage bushy growth.

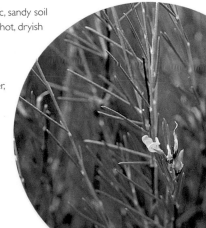

- Harvest small sprigs in the second summer. Bruise, chop, wet and pile them in a mound to oxidize (ferment), then sun-dry the leaves.

Lore and traditional uses
- The Bushmen and Khoi people of South Africa traditionally use rooibos to improve digestive disorders and treat irritated skin.

Enhancing mind and spirit
- To relieve stress, enjoy 3 cups rooibos leaf infusion (see first preparation, right), daily.

Caring for your body
- To benefit from rooibos's immune-boosting antioxidants, drink up to 3 cups rooibos leaf infusion (see first preparation, right), daily.
- To soothe tired eyes, soak two small pieces of gauze in cooled rooibos leaf infusion (see first preparation, right) and place one piece over each eye for 10 minutes.
- To relieve irritated skin, apply a rooibos compress (see second preparation, right) until the compress cools. Repeat frequently.

Core benefits

Boosts immunity

Mineral-rich

Rejuvenates the skin

Preparations

Infusion: 1 tsp dried rooibos leaves in 1 cup water. Standard method (p.20).

Compress: Use double-strength, hand-hot infusion (2 tsp dried rooibos leaves in 1 cup just-boiled water). Standard method (p.23).

95

Astragalus *Astragalus membranaceus*

Astragalus root is hailed as the most powerful immune-boosting herb in nature. The root increases the body's numbers of killer T-cells and antibodies, and enhances its production of a virus-fighting protein called interferon. Studies show that, in cancer patients, astragalus root can restore immune function in compromised cells. You can benefit from all astragalus's health-giving properties by taking the root in a pleasant-tasting decoction, or by adding slices of astragalus root to savoury recipes.

Plant type:
Hardy perennial

Description: 30cm (1ft) high by 30cm (1ft) wide; yellow pea-like flowers

Native habitat: Cool temperate; Mongolia

Parts of plant used: Roots

Growing and harvesting
- Requires a dry, well-drained soil in a sunny position.
- Sow fresh seeds in autumn in a cold frame; or, in the spring, soak dried seeds for 24 hours and then sow. (Germination can take four to nine weeks.)
- Once the plants are between four and seven years old, harvest roots in late autumn. Use fresh, or leave to dry.

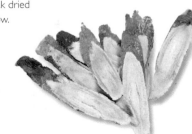

Lore and traditional uses
- Astragalus appears in the Chinese herbal the *Pen Tsao Ching* (100CE) as a "kingly" herb to enhance the entire body (see p.19).

Enhancing mind and spirit
- To strengthen *chi*, the building block of all spiritual and physical energy, drink ½ cup astragalus decoction (see first preparation, right), as required.

Caring for your body
- To strengthen immunity and tone the entire body, use sliced astragalus root in soups and stews and sprinkle powdered root on cereals.
- If you suffer from frequent colds or upper respiratory infections, such as bronchitis, take 1 tsp astragalus tincture (see second preparation, right) in a little water up to three times daily, for as long as required.
- To increase bloodflow to the skin and clear toxins from the body, drink a wine glassful of astragalus decoction (see first preparation, right) three times daily, as required.

Core benefits
Antiviral

Enhances body systems

Detoxifying

Preparations

Decoction: 30g (1oz) dried or 60g (2oz) fresh astragalus root in 750ml (1½ pints) water. Standard method (p.20).

Tincture: 200g (7oz) dried or 400g (14oz) fresh astragalus root in 1 litre (2 pints) vodka-water mix. Standard method (p.20).

Echinacea *Echinacea angustifolia*

The purple daisy flowers of this prairie herb will attract a host of bees and butterflies to your garden. Therapeutically, antibiotic and antiviral echinacea can kickstart the body's defences into high gear to stop a cold or the flu in its tracks. However, the herb's effectiveness slows down with continuous use, so use it primarily at the first signs of illness. Echinacea's roots have the most potent healing powers, although the leaves are effective, too.

Plant type:
Hardy perennial

Description: 1m (3ft) high by 45cm (1½ft) wide; red–purple flowers

Native habitat: Cool temperate; C North America

Parts of plant used: Roots, leaves, stems

Growing and harvesting
- Prefers rich, moist, well-drained soil in full sun.
- Grow from seed in a warm place. Plant out in spring.
- Harvest roots in autumn once the plant is two to four years old. Dry in shade.

Lore and traditional uses
- North American Plains Indians value echinacea to treat conditions as diverse as snake bites and fevers.

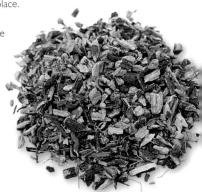

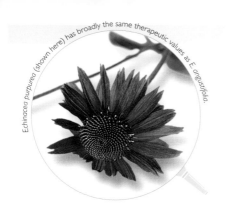

Echinacea purpurea (shown here) has broadly the same therapeutic values as E. angustifolia.

Enhancing mind and spirit

- To strengthen your healing energy, drink a wine glassful of echinacea decoction (see first preparation, right).

Caring for your body

- To halt an infection, every three to four hours during the first 24 hours of illness take up to three size 00 capsules filled with powdered echinacea root (see p.21), or 1½ tsp echinacea tincture (see second preparation, right) in a little water. Then, switch to astragalus (see pp.96–7).
- To relieve insect bites and stings, apply 1 drop echinacea tincture (see second preparation, right) to the area, as required.

Preparations

Decoction: 30g (1oz) dried echinacea root in 750ml (1½ pints) water. Standard method (p.20).

Tincture: 200g (7oz) dried echinacea root in 1 litre (2 pints) vodka-water mix. Standard method (p.20).

Licorice *Glycyrrhiza glabra*

Known in China as the "grandfather of herbs", licorice has been used medicinally all over the world for 4,000 years. In Traditional Chinese Medicine, licorice root is one of the "kingly" herbs (see p.19), and helps balance and regulate all body functions and stimulates immune cells to attack invading pathogens. Don't take more than 20g (¾oz) licorice root a day and avoid it altogether if you have high blood pressure.

Plant type:
Perennial

Description: 1m (3ft) high by 1m (3ft) wide; pale blue flowers

Native habitat: All temperate; Eurasia

Parts of plant used: Roots

Growing and harvesting

- Grow from runners (shoots that grow along the ground) that are 15cm (6in) long with a bud. In spring, plant runners 10cm (4in) deep in rich, fine, moist soil (not clay) in full sun.
- Keep roots moist during the growing season, but hot and dry in late summer to develop sweetness.
- Fertilize well and pick flowers as they start to grow, to improve root quality.
- Once the plant is three to four years old, harvest roots in autumn, and dry.

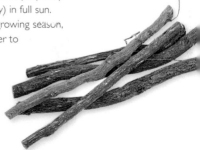

Lore and traditional uses

- In Egypt, during the time of the pharaohs, licorice water was a popular drink, probably because of its sweet taste.
- In ancient Rome, soldiers ate licorice to improve their energy and stamina for battle.
- Traditionally, brewers add licorice extract to porter and stout to give thickness and blackness to their brews.

Enhancing mind and spirit

- To clean the meridians and allow *chi* to flow smoothly (see p.18), chew fresh licorice root.

Caring for your body

- To ease a sore throat, drink a wine glassful of licorice decoction (see first preparation, right) three times daily, as required.
- To ease bronchial or asthmatic coughs, take 1–2 tsp licorice syrup (see second preparation, right) three times daily for two weeks. See a herbalist if the cough persists.
- To help neutralize toxins in the body, chew fresh licorice root.

Core benefits

Antimicrobial

Soothes respiration

Stimulates immunity

Preparations

Decoction: Simmer 3 tsp pieces of peeled, bruised licorice root, or 3 tsp licorice root powder, in 750ml (1½ pints) water for 10 minutes. Strain.

Syrup: Add 500ml (1 pint) honey to 500ml (1 pint) hot licorice root decoction (see above) and stir until dissolved. Cool and refrigerate (it will keep indefinitely).

Goldenseal *Hydrastis canadensis*

Said to be among the five top-selling herbal products in the USA, goldenseal's medicinal root is an antibiotic against bacteria and fungi, activates infection-fighting macrophage cells in the body, and improves blood supply to the spleen, which filters our blood to remove impurities. Contrary to modern myth, it will not mask a positive drugs test. Check with a medical herbalist before using goldenseal and avoid it altogether during pregnancy. Never use this herb for more than a week at a time.

Growing and harvesting
- Prefers to grow in a rich, moist, loamy soil in two-thirds shade.
- Grow from seed or from a root piece with a growing bud.
- Harvest roots in the second autumn. Use fresh, or dry.

Lore and traditional uses
- Native Americans used goldenseal root to treat infection-related inflammation in the respiratory, digestive and genito-urinary tracts.

Plant type:
Hardy perennial

Description: 30cm (1ft) high by 25cm (10in) wide; greenish-white flowers

Native habitat: Coniferous forest; Canada

Parts of plant used:
Roots

Preparations

Decoction: 30g (1oz) dried or 60g (2oz) fresh goldenseal root in 1 litre (2 pints) water. Standard method (p.20).

Tincture: 200g (7oz) dried or 400g (14oz) fresh goldenseal root in 1 litre (2 pints) vodka-water mix. Standard method (p.20).

Enhancing mind and spirit
- To counter mental or emotional fatigue, drink goldenseal decoction (see first preparation, left) as often as you like.

Caring for your body
- To treat mouth ulcers, gum disease and sore throats, gargle with 1 tsp goldenseal tincture (see second preparation, left) in a glass of warm water three times daily.
- For vaginal thrush or itching, douche with 1 tsp goldenseal decoction (see first preparation, left) in ½ cup water.
- To ease skin inflammation, especially in eczema or measles, bathe the affected areas with 1 tsp goldenseal tincture (see second preparation, left) in ½ cup water.
- For nail infections, apply a paste of 10 drops goldenseal tincture mixed with ½ tsp each vitamin E oil and honey.

Core benefits

Strengthens immunity

Soothes sinuses

Topical antiseptic

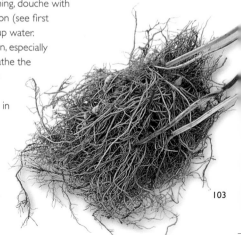

Oregano *Origanum vulgare*

The glorious springtime drifts of oregano's pink flowers on the hillsides of Greece earned this herb the name "Joy of the Mountain". Although oregano is probably best known for the fresh peppery leaves that flavour Italian pizza, Mexican enchiladas and bouquet garni, Polish research indicates that oregano has the strongest immune-boosting power of 70 tested herbs, including goldenseal (see pp.102–3).

Growing and harvesting
- Prefers dry, well-drained soil in a warm, sunny position.
- Sow seeds in early spring at 10–13°C (50–55°F) and only just cover with soil.
- Divide plant in spring or autumn and take cuttings in midsummer.
- Harvest whole plant (excluding roots) in late summer, and hang in small bunches to dry.

Lore and traditional uses
- The ancient Egyptians considered oregano sacred to Osiris, god of the dead, and wove it into ritual crowns and wreaths.

Plant type:
Hardy perennial

Description: 60cm (2ft) high by 75cm (2½ft) wide; small leaves

Native habitat: Warm temperate; Mediterranean

Parts of plant used: Leaves, flowers, essential oil (from leaves and small flowers)

Preparations

Triple-strength infusion: 3 tsp dried or 6 tsp fresh oregano leaves in 1 cup just-boiled water. Standard method (p.20).

Triple-strength infused oil: Use the infused-oil standard method (see p.23). Then, drain the oil (squeeze it from the leaves, too). Repeat the standard method using the drained oil, but fresh leaves, twice more.

- The ancient Greeks took this herb as an antidote to poison.

Enhancing mind and spirit

- To stimulate the throat *chakra* (see p.17) to gain emotional strength, massage 2 drops oregano leaf infused oil (see p.23) into your throat in a circle that goes clockwise to your left. Tap gently in the centre for a few seconds.

Caring for your body

- To stop a sore throat fast, gargle with and then drink 1 cup triple-strength oregano leaf infusion (see first preparation, left), or with 4 drops oregano triple-strength infused oil (see second preparation, left) in a cup of water, every two hours, between four and six times daily, until the sore throat has gone.
- To treat candida and ensuing infections on the nails or skin, apply a few drops oregano leaf infused oil (see p.23) to the affected areas three times daily until the candida has gone.

Core benefits

Kills pathogens

Antiparasitic

Fights candida

105

Elder *Sambucus nigra*

This easy-to-grow tree, with its muscatel-scented flowers, has been called a "complete medicine chest", because its leaves, flowers and berries all have therapeutic properties. Rising stars in the immune-boosting firmament, elderberries are extremely rich in antioxidants and a more potent antiviral than echinacea (see pp.98–9) – preliminary tests show that they are effective against the virus that causes Avian flu.

Plant type: Hardy, deciduous, shrubby tree

Description: 3.5m (12ft) tall by 3.5m (12ft) wide; cream flowers; dark berries

Native habitat: Cool temperate; Europe, SW Asia

Parts of plant used: Leaves, flowers, berries

Growing and harvesting
- Prefers moist, loamy soil in sun.
- Propagate from seeds or cuttings.
- Flowers in late spring, with fruits in early autumn.
- Collect flower heads in late spring; berries when heads tip downward. Use fresh, or dry.

Lore and traditional uses
- According to Danish lore, if you want to see the King of Fairyland, stand under an elder on midsummer's eve.

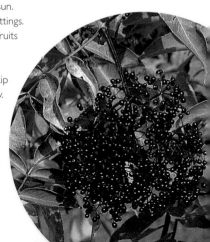

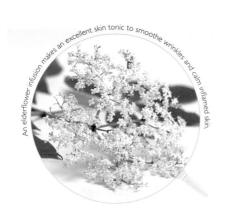

An elderflower infusion makes an excellent skin tonic to smoothe wrinkles and calm inflamed skin.

Enhancing mind and spirit

- To soothe frayed nerves, drink elderflower infusion (see first preparation, right).
- To ease nervous headaches, steam-iron some elder leaves and apply them hot to your brow.

Caring for your body

- To relieve feverish colds, take 1 cup elderberry infusion (see first preparation, right) three times daily.
- To soothe sunburn, wash the sore skin with cooled elderflower infusion (see first preparation, right) twice daily.
- For chilblains and chapped skin, apply elderflower cream (see second preparation, right), as required.

Preparations

Infusion: Use flowers or berries as appropriate: 1½ tsp dried or 3 tsp fresh elderflowers or 1 tsp dried or 2 tsp fresh elderberries in 1 cup just-boiled water. Standard method (p.20).

Elderflower cream: Melt 25g (1oz) beeswax. Add 8 tsp infused elderflower oil and 2 tsp elderflower tincture (p.20); strain, stir and press into a clean jar.

Schisandra *Schisandra chinensis*

The Chinese call the berries of this forest vine the Fruit of Five Flavours, as they possess all five basic tastes: bitter, sweet, pungent, salty and sour (see p.18). Together, these "tastes" help balance the whole body for overall well-being. This benefit is mirrored in Western herbalism, in which schisandra berries are said to boost immunity and offer a general healing tonic.

Growing and harvesting

- Grow in a rich, well-drained, slightly acidic-to-neutral soil, in sun to light shade.
- In autumn pre-soak seeds for 12 hours in warm water; grow plants in a greenhouse for one year (germination is difficult and you'll need male and female seeds unless you have the variety 'Eastern Prince'). Or grow from softwood cuttings taken in summer.
- Pick berries in summer. Use fresh, or sun-dry.

Lore and traditional uses

- In ancient China, uses for schisandra included increasing energy, treating fatigue, suppressing a cough and increasing sexual vigour.

Main type: Hardy deciduous climber

Description: Up to 8m (27ft) long; fragrant white flowers; red berries

Native habitat: Cool temperate; N China, Korea

Parts of plant used: Berries

Preparations

Tonic wine: 100g (3½oz) dried or 200g (7oz) fresh schisandra berries in 1 litre (2 pints) red wine. Standard method (p.22).

Tincture: 200g (7oz) dried or 400g (14oz) fresh schisandra berries in 1 litre (2 pints) vodka-water mix. Standard method (p.20).

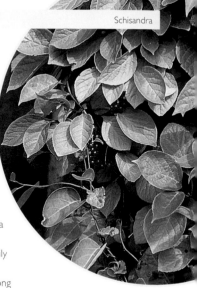

Enhancing mind and spirit

- To enhance the "Three Treasures" (see p.18) of *chi* (vital force), *jing* (nutritive essence) and *shen* (spirit), juice fresh schisandra berries as required, then dilute them to taste in water or another juice of your choice, and drink.
- To reduce mental confusion, drink a sherry glassful of schisandra tonic wine (see first preparation, left) daily before a meal.
- For a sustaining energy boost on long journeys, eat dried schisandra berries.

Caring for your body

- To boost the immune system and strengthen the liver against infection, eat whole fresh or dried berries, including the seed, regularly.
- To help normalize blood-sugar levels and to increase vitality, take ½–1 tsp schisandra tincture (see second preparation, left) in a little water or juice, three times daily.

Core benefits

Protects the liver

Modulates stress

Boosts vitality

Pau d'arco *Tabebuia impetiginosa*

With its stunning purple flowers, the pau d'arco tree is popular in tropical gardens. It has hardwearing insect- and weather-resistant timber used to make structures such as the famous boardwalk in Atlantic City. The tree's healing qualities come from the *inner bark*, which is antibacterial, antiviral and antifungal. Of pau d'arco's 20 or so active compounds, several have anti-tumour effects.

Plant type: Half-hardy deciduous tree

Description: 30m (100ft) tall by 8m (65ft) wide, purple trumpet flowers

Native habitat: Tropical rainforest; S America

Parts of plant used: Inner bark, heartwood (innermost trunk)

Growing and harvesting

- Grow from seeds or cuttings in well-drained, fertile soil in humid conditions and sun.
- Hardy to temperatures as low as -4°C (25°F), but protect during frosts.
- The inner bark is harvested from wild trees, which are usually cut for timber.

Lore and traditional uses

- Meaning "bow wood", pau d'arco was so called because the wood's

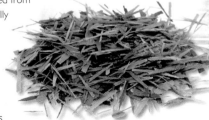

110

strength made it the perfect material for native hunters to make weapons with.
- In the 19th century, a Russian chemist created a pau d'arco toothpaste to stop tooth decay.

Enhancing mind and spirit
- To boost vigour, drink 1 cup pau d'arco decoction (see first preparation, right), three times daily.

Caring for your body
- For candida, take 1 size 00 capsule filled with powdered pau d'arco inner bark (see p.21), three times daily, and wear a tampon dipped in pau d'arco decoction (see first preparation, right), renewed twice daily for three days.
- For relief from flu, drink ½–1 cup pau d'arco decoction (see first preparation, right) two to four times daily.
- To heal warts, at bedtime soak a small piece of cotton wool in pau d'arco tincture (see second preparation, right) and fix over the wart using a plaster. Leave overnight. Repeat nightly until the wart disappears.

Core benefits

Antimicrobial

Fights tumours

Painkilling

Preparations

Decoction: 30g (1oz) pau d'arco inner bark chips in 750ml (1½ pints) water. Standard method (p.20).

Tincture: 200g (7oz) pau d'arco inner bark in 1 litre (2 pints) vodka-water mix. Standard method (p.20).

CHAPTER 4

Protective Herbs

The herbs in this chapter have been chosen because they have a special protective power over some aspect of our well-being – physical, mental, emotional, spiritual and even environmental.

Many of these herbs protect a particular part of the body or protect the body from a particular kind of illness. For example, fennel protects the liver; bilberry, the eyes; and stevia, against obesity. Sweet wormwood has an incredible ability to protect against new strains of malaria; lady's mantle nurtures all aspects of womanhood, including fertility (early alchemists and herbalists used dew drops from its leaves in healing elixirs for women); and feverfew reduces migraines (an old wives' tale verified by scientific research).

Other herbs, such as thyme, are protective because they have strong antimicrobial properties. As well as providing antibacterial, antifungal and

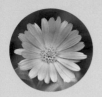
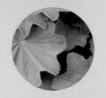
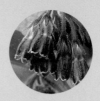

antiviral protection for the body, these herbs are useful in the home as natural cleaners and disinfectants.

Protective herbs can influence the wider environment, too. I have included neem because the tree itself helps protect humanity from global warming. Similarly, comfrey can be made into an organic fertilizer, reducing the need for us to use chemicals on our crops. Both these herbs also extend

their protective qualities to the body – neem boosts the immune system and comfrey speeds cell renewal.

Finally, the chapter includes herbs that help protect the mind and spirit as well as the body. Calendula is pure feel-good factor in a flower (and has amazing skin-protecting properties), while sweet violet helps calm fiery emotions, restoring a sense of equilibrium and gentleness to the spirit.

Lady's mantle *Alchemilla mollis*

The botanical name for lady's mantle, *Alchemilla* – from the Arab *alkemelych* (alchemy) – means "little magical one", which reflects this herb's protective and curative powers. Lady's mantle is taken to regulate periods, ease menopause and clear inflammation of the female organs. In his *Complete Herbal* of 1653, English herbalist Nicholas Culpeper wrote that drinking and applying lady's mantle could shrink and firm bosoms "that be too great and flaggie". Avoid using this herb during pregnancy.

Plant type:
Hardy perennial

Description: 60cm (2ft) high by 70cm (2½ft) wide; clusters of yellow flowers

Native habitat: Cool temperate; Europe, N Asia

Parts of plant used: Leaves, roots

Growing and harvesting

- Prefers a rich, well-drained, moist soil in full sun or partial shade.
- Sow seeds in spring; or divide plants in spring or autumn.
- Harvest fresh leaves as needed, or for drying during flowering. Dig up two-year-old roots in autumn.
- Cut stalks to the base after blooming to encourage new autumn leaves.

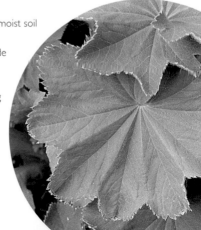

Lore and traditional uses

- In the 15th and 16th centuries, lady's mantle was used on European battlefields for its wound-healing properties.
- Lady's mantle is planted on Alpine pastures to increase the milk production of grazing cows.

Enhancing mind and spirit

- For deep spiritual peace after an emotional shock, put 2 drops lady's mantle flower essence (see pp.34–5) in a glass of water and sip throughout the day.

Caring for your body

- For menstrual problems, take 1 cup lady's mantle leaf infusion (see first preparation, right), three times daily as needed.
- For a breast-firming treatment, massage the breasts twice daily, every day, with lady's mantle root infused oil (see p.23).
- To reduce puffy eyes, make a lady's mantle compress (see second preparation, right). Place it as hot as is comfortable over your closed eyes and rest for 20 minutes.

Core benefits

Regulates menstruation

Astringent

Anti-inflammatory

Preparations

Infusion: 1 tsp dried or 2 tsp fresh lady's mantle leaves in 1 cup just-boiled water. Standard method (p.20).

Compress: Soak some gauze in double-strength lady's mantle leaf infusion (2 tsp dried or 4 tsp fresh leaves in 1 cup water). Standard method (p.23).

Sweet wormwood *Artemisia annua*

Sweet wormwood is a herb that could save a million lives a year. Used for decades by the Chinese army to prevent and treat malaria, this herb contains a compound called artemisinin, which is the only known treatment for drug-resistant strains of malaria. In trials, artemisinin is showing promise as a possible anti-cancer compound, too. The compound is found in specialized cells that protrude from the surface of the plant's leaves, stems and flowers. Avoid sweet wormwood during pregnancy.

Growing and harvesting

- Grows easily, but prefers a well-drained, loamy soil and sunny position.
- Sow seeds *in situ* in late spring
- Harvest leaves in summer, before the plant comes into flower (from August to September). Use fresh, or dry.

Lore and traditional uses

- In Traditional Chinese Medicine, sweet wormwood leaf infusion has been used for more than 1,500 years to treat fevers.

Plant type:
Annual

Description: 2.5m (8ft) high by 60cm (2ft) wide; panicles of yellow flowers

Native habitat: Cool temperate; Asia, SE Europe

Parts of plant used: Flowers, leaves, stems, seeds, essential oil (from seeds)

Preparations

Infusion: 1 tsp dried or 2 tsp fresh sweet wormwood leaves in 1 cup just-boiled water. Standard method (p.20). Sweeten if necessary.

Compress: Soak some gauze in hand-hot, double-strength sweet wormwood leaf infusion (1½ tsp dried or 6 tsp fresh leaves in 1 cup water). Standard method (p.23).

- In Indo-China, sweet wormwood treats jaundice, dysentery and skin complaints.

Enhancing mind and spirit
- To cool strong emotions, such as anger, place a few drops of sweet wormwood leaf infused oil (see p.23) on a tissue and inhale.

Caring for your body
- For an emergency anti-malarial treatment, take 1 cup sweet wormwood leaf infusion (see first preparation, left) every six hours, for seven days. (And seek medical advice as soon as possible.)
- To treat coughs, colds and sinus problems, inhale the vapour from a cup of hot sweet wormwood leaf infusion (see first preparation, left) for 10 minutes, three times daily, until better.
- To soothe sore or inflamed insect bites or stings, make a sweet wormwood compress (see second preparation, left) and apply it to the affected areas as often as necessary.

Core benefits
Kills malaria parasite
Aids respiratory system
Anti-cancer

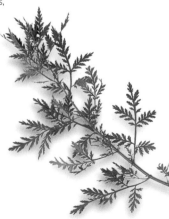

Neem *Azadirachta indica*

Resilient against global warming, a non-toxic pesticide and an air-purifier, neem is nature's answer to 21st-century problems. The plant's leaves and essential oil are antifungal, antiviral and antibacterial. They help lower blood sugar, blood pressure and bad cholesterol and stimulate immunity. Neem bark and leaf extract show anti-cancer and anti-AIDS potential.

Plant type:
Tender evergreen tree

Description: 16m (53ft) tall by 18m (60ft) wide; fragrant white flowers

Native habitat: Tropical dry; East Indies, Africa

Parts of plant used:
Leaves, flowers, bark, wood, seeds, essential oil (from seeds)

Growing and harvesting
- Requires hot, dry, sunny conditions. Dies in frost or on waterlogged sites.
- Sow seed that is less than six months old in warm sun, or plant root suckers *in situ*.
- Harvest leaves any time; seeds after three to five years.

Lore and traditional uses
- In India, neem gained divine status when drops from the Elixir of Immortality fell onto the neem tree.
- Indian women use leaves to protect rice from pests.

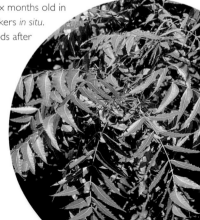

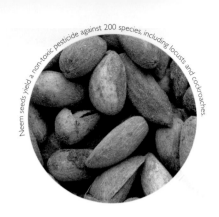

Neem seeds yield a non-toxic pesticide against 200 species, including locusts and cockroaches.

Enhancing mind and spirit

• Follow a Hindu proverb: plant three neem trees to improve your karma.

Caring for your body

• To improve dental health, rub neem twigs over your gums and teeth, twice daily.

• To treat a wart, acne or eczema, apply neem balm (see first preparation, right), morning and evening, until your skin has recovered.

• To treat candida, make a strong neem leaf infusion (see second preparation, right). While hot, drink 1 cup; then douche with ½ cup at room temperature and insert a tampon just dipped in the remainder (replace three times daily). Repeat until the infection has cleared.

Preparations

Balm: Place 3 tsp neem pressed seed oil (available to buy), 3 tsp olive oil and 1¼ tsp beeswax in a bowl over a pan of simmering water. Stir until melted. Cool, stir in 5 drops lavender essential oil. Store in a lidded pot.

Strong infusion: Place 50 fresh or dry neem leaves in 500ml (1 pint) just-boiled water, cover. Stand for 24 hours. Strain.

119

Calendula *Calendula officinalis*

Sunshine in a flower, this cheerful, hardy annual is so often in bloom that it gives the impression of being in flower on the first day – the "calend" – of every month. Valued by the ancient Egyptians as a rejuvenating herb, calendula now finds its way into many skin creams where it provides antiseptic, antifungal and antioxidant properties. In France, clinical trials have found that, applied topically, calendula is 50 percent more successful than conventional drugs at reducing skin damage caused by radiation treatment for breast-cancer patients.

Plant type:
Hardy annual

Description: 60cm (2ft) high by 45cm (1½ft) wide; deep golden flowers

Native habitat: Warm temperate; Mediterranean

Parts of plant used: Flowers, leaves

Growing and harvesting

- Will succeed in any well-drained soil and sunny position.
- Sow seeds *in situ* from spring to early summer.
- Harvest flowers when fully open; leaves any time. Use either part fresh or dried, but dry the flowers quickly after harvesting, or infuse the petals in oil.

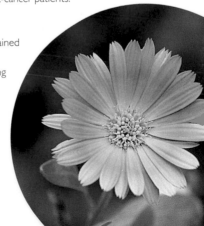

Lore and traditional uses
- According to medieval lore, if a girl touches the petals of calendula flowers with her bare feet, she will understand birdsong.
- During the American Civil War, doctors used calendula leaves to treat open wounds.

Enhancing mind and spirit
- To realize dreams and protect yourself from evil as you sleep, sprinkle a handful of calendula petals under your bed.
- To release nervousness, add 2 cups calendula petal infusion (see first preparation, right) to a warm bath and soak for 20 minutes.

Caring for your body
- To soothe cracked or chapped skin, or nipples that are sore from breastfeeding, apply a few drops infused calendula leaf or petal oil (see p.23) twice daily, as necessary.
- To heal a baby's nappy rash, or to treat leg ulcers, varicose veins, bed sores or bruises, apply calendula ointment (see second preparation, right) three times daily.

Core benefits

Protects the skin

Antimicrobial

Reduces inflammation

Preparations

Infusion: 1–2 tsp dried calendula petals in 1 cup just-boiled water. Standard method (p.20).

Ointment: Heat 1 cup infused calendula oil (see p.23) in a pan until warm. Remove from the heat and combine with 30g (1oz) melted beeswax. Stir until cool. Pour into clean jars, secure the lids, and label. Store for up to 1 year.

Fennel *Foeniculum vulgare*

All parts of this tall, feathery herb have a clean, aniseed flavour, and children often love to pick the young stems and nibble them as "licorice celery". Fennel's seeds, leaves and stems are well known for their ability to aid the digestive system, but new research indicates that fennel may also offer protection for the liver, helping repair this organ following alcohol damage. Try sprouting the seeds for a novel addition to salads.

Plant type:
Hardy evergreen perennial

Description: 2m (6ft) high by 1m (3ft) wide; tiny yellow flower clusters

Native habitat: All temperate; Europe

Parts of plant used: Seeds, flowers, leaves, stems, roots

Growing and harvesting

- There are green and bronze leaf varieties available – both will succeed in most soils and prefer a sunny position.
- Sow seeds in spring. Or propagate by dividing plants any time.
- Harvest leaves any time, then use fresh, or freeze for later use; pick flowers in late summer and use fresh. Collect seeds when ripe in autumn; dry for storage.

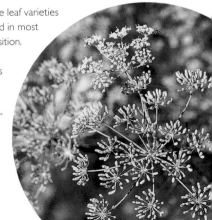

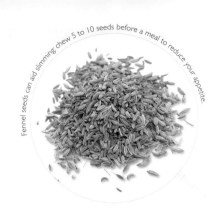

Fennel seeds can aid slimming: chew 5 to 10 seeds before a meal to reduce your appetite.

Reduces bloating

Slimming aid

Eases digestion

Lore and traditional uses

• Fennel was one of the nine herbs sacred to the Anglo-Saxons for its power to protect against evil.

Enhancing mind and spirit

• To release negative energy, put 2 drops fennel flower essence (see pp.34–5) in water and sip while meditating on the plant.

Caring for your body

• To relieve indigestion, take 1 cup fennel seed infusion (see first preparation, right) up to three times daily, as required.

• For a deep skin cleanse, try a fennel steam inhalation (see second preparation, right).

Preparations

Infusion: Crush ½ tsp dried fennel seeds and infuse in 1 cup just-boiled water for 10 minutes. Strain.

Inhalation: Place 2 tsp crushed fennel seeds or 2 handfuls fresh fennel leaves in a bowl containing 3 litres (6 pints) boiling water. Standard method (p.22).

Stevia *Stevia rebaudiana*

Like a gift from the gods, stevia is 10 to 15 times sweeter than sugar yet is calorie-free and does not raise blood-sugar levels. Studies suggest that the herb improves insulin sensitivity and may help reverse diabetes, although in some countries these findings are treated with caution. Researchers at Purdue University in Indiana have concluded that stevia inhibits the development of dental plaque, and may help prevent tooth cavities. Stevia plants vary in their sweetness and aftertaste, so try to find cuttings from known high-quality mother plants.

Growing and harvesting
- Prefers a well-drained, loamy soil in partial shade, but will tolerate most soils.
- Surface-sow seeds, and – to speed germination – maintain a temperature of 25°C (77°F) or higher.
- For the sweetest leaves, harvest them before the first frost or as soon as flowering begins, whichever comes first.
- Cut the entire plant 15cm (6in) above the ground. Hang it upside down to dry.

Plant type:
Half-hardy perennial

Description: 80cm (2½ft) high by 45cm (1½ft) wide; white tubular flowers

Native habitat: All tropical; S America

Parts of plant used: Leaves

Preparations

Syrup: Boil 2 cups water in a pan. Lower the heat and add 3 tbsp dried stevia leaves. Boil again for 3 minutes. Cool, filter, bottle and refrigerate.

Infusion: 1 tsp stevia powder or 2 tsp fresh stevia leaves in 1 cup just-boiled water. Standard method (p.20).

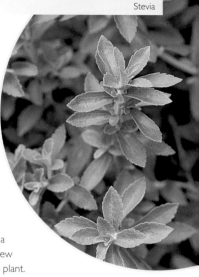

Lore and traditional uses

- In South America, stevia is known as the "honey leaf" and sold as an aid to people with diabetes and hypoglycemia.
- During World-War-II rationing, the English grew stevia as a sugar substitute.

Enhancing mind and spirit

- To avoid an emotional craving for sweet food, add 2 stevia leaves to a regular cup of tea, and drink; or chew a fresh leaf taken directly from the plant.

Caring for your body

- As an aid to effective weight-management, replace sugar and artificial sweetners with stevia syrup (see first preparation, left) in hot drinks and in cooking.
- To improve the health of the teeth, gargle with a cooled stevia infusion (see second preparation, left) twice daily, morning and evening, as required.

Core benefits
Aids weight loss
Balances blood sugar
Reduces tooth decay

Comfrey *Symphytum officinale*

In the 19th century, British smallholder Henry Doubleday championed comfrey as an organic fertilizer, because the leaf contains the three key elements that make up many chemical fertilizers: nitrogen, potassium and phosphorous. It also contains calcium and the compound allantoin, which speeds cell renewal in the body's muscles, bones and connective tissue. High amounts of chlorophyll in comfrey leaves promote healing and purify the blood. Avoid the internal use of the roots; or of any part of the plant if you suffer from liver disease.

Plant type:
Hardy perennial

Description: 20cm (8in) high by 60cm (2ft) wide; white or mauve flowers

Native habitat: Cool temperate; N Europe

Parts of plant used: Leaves, stems, roots, flowers

Growing and harvesting

- Tolerates most soils and light shade.
- Grow from roots or offsets taken any time except during frost. Or divide mature plants.
- Use fresh leaves any time, but to dry, harvest in early summer before flowering. Pick flowers in summer and two-year-old roots in autumn. Use fresh, or dry.

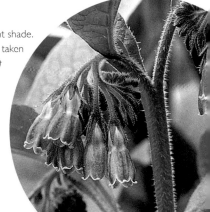

Lore and traditional uses
- Dioscorides, a Greek physician writing in 50CE, prescribed comfrey to heal broken bones.
- Medieval women took a comfrey bath to repair the hymen and recreate "virginity".

Enhancing mind and spirit
- To activate the sacral *chakra* (see p.17), add 2 drops comfrey flower essence (see pp.34–5) to a glass of water and sip throughout the day.

Caring for your body
- For rough skin patches, minor cuts or aching joints, apply comfrey salve (see first preparation, right) to the affected areas.
- To treat gum disease, gargle with cooled comfrey leaf infusion (see second preparation, right) three times daily, as required.

Special tip
To make comfrey fertilizer, fill a bucket with fresh comfrey leaves, then cover with water and a lid. Leave for six weeks. Before using, dilute 1 part comfrey liquid to 15 parts water.

Core benefits

Heals bone and tendons

Heals wounds

Relieves congestion

Preparations

Salve: Melt ½ cup infused comfrey leaf or root oil, ½ cup infused calendula petal oil (see p.23) and 1½ tsp beeswax in a pan. Cool, then add 6 drops each lavender and thyme essential oils. Stir and bottle for up to 1 year.

Infusion: 1 tsp dried comfrey leaves in 1 cup just-boiled water. Standard method (p.20).

Feverfew *Tanacetum parthenium*

Modern herbalists use feverfew to reduce the frequency and severity of migraines. Taken cumulatively, the herb relaxes the smooth muscles of the neck and spine to reduce spasm, and inhibits the secretion of serotonin, a compound implicated in migraines and rheumatoid arthritis. Historically, feverfew has also been used to reduce fevers, cleanse the uterus and expel worms. Avoid taking feverfew if you are pregnant or on blood-thinning drugs.

Plant type: Hardy, evergreen perennial

Description: 60cm (2ft) high by 30cm (1ft) wide; scalloped leaves

Native habitat: Cool temperate; Eurasia, SE Europe

Parts of plant used: Leaves, stems, flowers

Growing and harvesting

- Grows easily in most soils (even poor soils and dry conditions), but needs sun.
- Sow seeds in spring in a greenhouse. Only just cover with soil and don't allow to dry out. Or propagate by dividing plants in spring.
- Pick leaves any time; harvest flowering tops in midsummer.

Lore and traditional uses

- In the 17th century, European herbalists sold a feverfew skin lotion intended to remove blemishes and freckles.

Preparations

Infusion: 1 tsp dried or 2 tsp fresh feverfew leaves in 1 cup just-boiled water. Standard method (p.20). (For a weak infusion, use ½ tsp dried or 1 tsp fresh leaves in 1 cup water.)

Poultice: Sauté 2 handfuls fresh feverfew leaves in a little oil, and apply hand-hot to the area.

- Feverfew leaves are used in dried posies and sachets of dried plants to deter moths.

Enhancing mind and spirit

- To overcome melancholy, drink 1 cup feverfew leaf infusion (see first preparation, left) up to three times daily, as required.

Caring for your body

- To prevent migraines, eat 2–4 small feverfew leaves daily (on bread if, eaten on their own, the leaves irritate your mouth lining). The effect is cumulative, so do this for six months.
- To ease dragging period pain, take 1 cup weak feverfew leaf infusion (see first preparation, left) up to three times daily, as needed.
- To soothe digestive spasms, apply a feverfew poultice (see second preparation, left) to the abdomen, as required.

Core benefits

Relieves migraines

Regulates menstruation

Anti-rheumatic

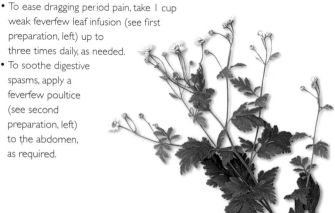

Thyme *Thymus vulgaris*

Thyme, which is antibacterial, antifungal and antiseptic, is one of nature's protective superstars. The key to its efficacy lies in its essential oil. In the 1960s, French biochemist Jean Valnet proved that thyme essential oil was better than several other essential oils at destroying microbes. Its main active compound is thymol, which is often used as a hospital antiseptic and in mouthwashes. However, thyme is eight times more powerful when taken as a "whole herb", which enables all its constituents to work in synergy. Avoid using thyme medicinally during pregnancy (although culinary uses are fine).

Growing and harvesting

- Prefers light, well-drained, alkaline soil in sun; dislikes heavy, wet soils.
- In spring, surface-sow seeds in a greenhouse; but it is easiest to propagate from 8cm (3in) cuttings taken any time except winter.
- Pick leaves or sprigs any time to use fresh. Harvest for drying in late summer just before the flowers open. Dry quickly.

Plant type: Hardy evergreen small shrub

Description: 20cm (8 in) high by 30cm (1ft) wide; lilac summer flowers

Native habitat: Warm temperate; W Mediterranean

Parts of plant used: Flowers, leaves, stems, essential oil (from leaves)

Preparations

Infusion: 1 tsp dried or 2 tsp fresh thyme sprigs in 1 cup just-boiled water. Standard method (p.20).

Tincture: 200g (7oz) dried or 400g (14oz) fresh thyme leaves or sprigs in 1 litre (2 pints) vodka-water mix. Standard method (p.20).

Lore and traditional uses
- Egyptians used the antiseptic and preservative powers of thyme for embalming.
- In the Middle Ages, thyme tea was often taken for coughs, indigestion and intestinal worms.

Enhancing mind and spirit
- To cleanse and protect your home, burn a few sprigs of thyme and waft the aromatic smoke through the rooms.
- To stimulate memory and concentration, drink 1 cup thyme infusion (see first preparation, left) three times daily.

Caring for your body
- To treat a persistent cough and respiratory congestion, take 1 cup thyme infusion (see first preparation, left) up to three times daily, until your condition has improved.
- To relieve bad breath or gum disease, take 1 tsp thyme tincture (see second preparation, left) in a little water or juice three times daily.

Core benefits

Antimicrobial

Expectorant

Stimulates memory

Bilberry *Vaccinium myrtillus*

During World War II, pilots experienced improved night vision after eating bilberry jam. Since then, research indicates bilberry extract can protect your retina and improve its blood supply, preventing disorders such as macular degeneration, cataracts and glaucoma. Bilberry leaves are high in chromium, which helps regulate blood-sugar levels. The deep blue colour of the fruit indicates dense levels of anthocyanins (potent antioxidants that protect the body from free radicals) and cytikine, a protein that protects against cell aging.

Plant type: Hardy, low-growing shrub

Description: 60cm (2ft) high by 60cm (2ft) wide; pinky white flowers

Native habitat: Cool temperate; Eurasia, N America

Parts of plant used: Fruit, leaves

Growing and harvesting
- Prefers a peaty, well-drained, moist, acidic soil in sun or light shade.
- In late winter, surface-sow seeds in a greenhouse. Or propagate from cuttings taken in autumn.
- Use summer berries fresh, dry, or juiced then frozen. Harvest leaves in early autumn. Use fresh, or dry.

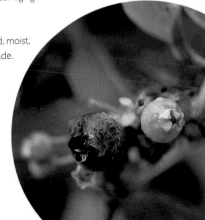

Lore and traditional uses
- In 16th-century England, Elizabethans made a medicinal drink called a "rob", a bilberry syrup sweetened with honey, to treat diarrhea.

Enhancing mind and spirit
- To bring luck and benevolence into your life, drink a small glass of bilberry juice daily.

Caring for your body
- For vision-related conditions, including macular degeneration, night blindness and diabetic retinopathy, take 1 cup bilberry decoction (see first preparation, right) three times daily, as necessary.
- To reduce varicose veins, drink 1 cup bilberry leaf infusion (see second preparation, right) three times daily for up to three weeks; break for a week, then resume if necessary.
- To reduce tiny thread veins and maintain the elasticity of your skin, drink 2 tsp bilberry juice four times daily, and apply bilberry lotion (see third preparation, right) every morning and evening.

Core benefits
Antioxidant

Supports vision

Strengthens circulation

Preparations

Decoction: Place 1 or 2 tsp mashed fresh bilberries in 1 cup water in a pan. Boil then simmer for 10 minutes; strain.

Infusion: 1 tsp dried or 2 tsp fresh bilberry leaves in 1 cup just-boiled water. Standard method (p.20).

Lotion: Mix 2 tbsp bilberry juice with 2 tbsp witch hazel.

Sweet violet *Viola odorata*

This pretty herald of spring features in medieval tapestries alongside dragons, knights and unicorns, to symbolize humility. The plant's leaves, flowers and rhizome all have medicinal, culinary, cosmetic and dye uses. They are high in vitamins A and C, and contain salicylic acid, which is used to make aspirin, confirming the herb's folk value for treating headaches, migraines and insomnia. A poultice of fresh sweet violet leaves has been used to treat skin conditions such as skin cancer for 2,000 years.

Plant type: Hardy, creeping evergreen perennial

Description: 10cm (4in) high by 45cm (1½ft) wide; sweetly scented flowers

Native habitat: Cool temperate; S, C and W Europe

Parts of plant used: Flowers, leaves, rhizome, essential oil (from leaves)

Growing and harvesting

- Prefers a moist, well-drained, humus-rich soil in dappled shade.
- Easiest to propagate from runners; detach in spring or autumn and replant. Or sow seeds in autumn.
- In leaf all year round; harvest any time; use fresh, or dry. Harvest flowers during spring and use fresh, or dry for later use.

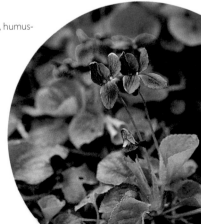

Lore and traditional uses

- Associated with the love-goddess Aphrodite, sweet violet was a symbol of fertility to the ancient Greeks, who used it in love potions.
- The ancient Romans welcomed spring with *violetum*, a sweet-violet wine.

Enhancing mind and spirit

- To moderate anger or anxiety, put a drop of sweet violet leaf essential oil on your wrists, temples and inner elbows, then meditate on your heart *chakra* (see p.17) for 10 minutes.

Caring for your body

- To reduce a headache or insomnia, take up to 3 cups sweet violet leaf infusion (see first preparation, right), as required.
- To moisturize dry skin, or to remove make-up, use sweet violet cream (see second preparation, right), as required.
- For a natural facial, stir a handful of sweet violet flowers into ½ cup live yogurt. Leave at room temperature overnight. Apply to your face and neck. Leave for 10 minutes; rinse off.

Preparations

Infusion: 1 tsp dried or 2 tsp fresh sweet violet leaves in 1 cup just-boiled water. Standard method (p.20).

Cream: Melt 25g (1oz) beeswax and 120ml (4fl oz) infused sweet violet oil (leaves and flowers; see p.23) in a bowl over a pan of simmering water. Remove from the heat and whisk until cooled. Pour into jars.

CHAPTER 5

Body Tonics

In the 1940s, Russian scientists took several groups of people suffering from prolonged stress and tested their responses to certain herbs, including ginseng, eleuthero and golden root. They found that these plants increase the body's ability to adapt to and cope with internal and external stresses.

Centuries earlier, the Chinese called a group of herbs with similar properties to these the "kingly" herbs (see p.19), but the Russians called their discoveries "adaptogens".

In cases of long-term stress, whether from a heavy workload or a chronic lack of sleep, adaptogens help the body recover faster and rebuild both mental and physical reserves. Adaptogens help keep stress under control and create within us the physical and mental agility for both a better and longer life. As well as ginseng, eleuthero and golden root,

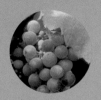
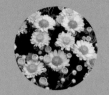
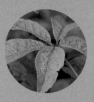

this chapter's adaptogens are maral root, dang shen and reishi mushroom. Use them whenever stress takes hold.

Adaptogens are not the only kinds of herb to provide us with body tonics. Other contributions come from the tea chrysanthemum, sage and the beautiful peony. In Africa, the kinkeliba tree provides a body tonic that not only energizes the body, but also induces restful and restorative sleep.

Herbs that help boost the circulation or protect the heart and blood are also useful body tonics. Hawthorn, goji berries, alfalfa and grape (in particular, red grape) score highly on these fronts. Sweet cicely helps right imbalances in the urinary, digestive and respiratory systems.

This chapter presents a range of extraordinary herbs to cherish, because they offer the nearest things we have to contemporary elixirs of life.

Tea chrysanthemum *Chrysanthemum × grandiflorum*

Legend claims that inhabitants of the Chinese village of Yeohyeon were known for their longevity. Always looking out for elixirs of life, some Taoist Masters went to investigate. They discovered the tea chrysanthemum growing along the village stream, adding its properties to the drinking water, and proclaimed it a longevity herb. Its cooling, antibiotic, antiviral properties reduce blood pressure, disperse toxins, improve brain function, pacify the liver, protect the body's cells and refresh the eyes.

Plant type:
Hardy perennial

Description: 1m (3ft) high by 60cm (2ft) wide; small yellow flowers

Native habitat: Cool temperate; E Asia, N Africa

Parts of plant used: Flowering tops

Growing and harvesting

- Prefers well-drained soil in a sunny position or part shade.
- Sow seeds *in situ* in spring or after midsummer; or take cuttings in late spring. (The plant often self-seeds.)
- This is a "short-day" plant: the longer nights of autumn induce flowering. Harvest floral heads and leave to dry in the sun.

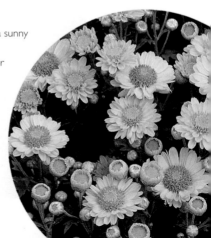

Lore and traditional uses

- In Japan, the Imperial seal features a 16-petalled chrysanthemum to symbolize longevity and joy.

Enhancing mind and spirit

- For a happy mood and calm heart, add ½ handful tea chrysanthemum petals to rice or oatmeal porridge while heating, and eat for breakfast each morning.
- To improve mental alertness, take 1 cup tea chrysanthemum flower infusion (see first preparation, right) up to three times daily.

Caring for your body

- To treat varicose veins, place a tea chrysanthemum compress (see second preparation, right) on the affected area every morning and evening.
- To relieve red, tired eyes, soak two small gauze squares in tea chrysanthemum flower infusion (see first preparation, right) and gently wring out. Lay one square over each eye and rest like that for 10 minutes.

Core benefits

Improves circulation

Stimulates mental focus

Antimicrobial

Preparations

Infusion: 1 tsp dried or 2 tsp fresh tea chrysanthemum flowers in 1 cup just-boiled water. Standard method (p.20).

Compress: Use double-strength, hand-hot flower infusion (2 tsp dried or 4 tsp fresh tea chrysanthemum flowers in 1 cup just-boiled water). Standard method (p.23).

Dang shen *Codonopsis pilosula*

This twining perennial herb has tuberous roots and oval or heart-shaped leaves that have a curious smell when crushed. Long stalks play host to pendulous pale green, purple-patterned bell-flowers. An adaptogen (see p.136), dang shen root benefits the whole body by boosting its stamina to withstand internal and external stresses. The root is able to stimulate the nervous system, increase mental alertness, lower blood pressure and strengthen immunity, and has been used to treat HIV.

Plant type: Hardy perennial climber

Description: Up to 1.5m (5ft) long; pale green flowers with purple pattern

Native habitat: Cool temperate; N China, Korea

Parts of plant used: Roots

Growing and harvesting

- Prefers a well-drained, light, fertile acid-to-neutral soil in full sun or partial shade.
- Surface sow seeds from spring to early summer in moist, acid compost. Keep in a greenhouse for first winter. Or propagate by dividing plants in spring.
- Once plants are more than three years old, harvest roots in autumn. Use fresh, or dry.

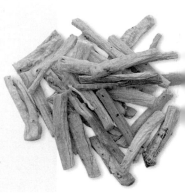

Lore and traditional uses

- Dang shen is one of the "four gentleman" in the Chinese energy tonic "soup of the four gentlemen". (The other three are the Chinese herbs fu ling, gan cao and bai zhu.)
- In Chinese medicine, dang shen treats breast cancer, asthma, diabetes, heart palpitations, memory or appetite loss, and insomnia.

Enhancing mind and spirit

- To strengthen *chi* (see p.18) and help cope with emotional stress, drink 1 cup dang shen decoction (see first preparation, right) up to three times daily for as long as required.

Caring for your body

- To stimulate immunity, increase both red- and white-blood-cell counts and reduce toxicity, take 1 tsp dang shen tincture (see second preparation, right) three times daily.
- To boost physical energy and improve stamina, drink 1 cup dang shen decoction (see first preparation, right) up to three times daily, as necessary.

Core benefits

Boosts vitality

Enhances brain function

Stimulates immunity

Preparations

Decoction: 30g (1oz) dried or 60g (2oz) fresh dang shen root in 750ml (1½ pints) water. Standard method (p.20).

Tincture: 200g (7oz) dried or 400g (14oz) fresh dang shen root in 1 litre (2 pints) vodka-water mix. Standard method (p.20).

141

Kinkeliba *Combretum micranthum*

While working in Gambia, I often noticed local lads taking handfuls of leaves from a wild kinkeliba bush: they boiled the leaves (over burners containing kinkeliba-wood charcoal) to make a syrupy green tea, which they drank as an energizing tonic. As well as its restorative properties, kinkeliba cleanses the blood, reduces stomach cramps and promotes deep, restful sleep. The plant is accredited with helping weight loss, and has been used cosmetically in a body-shaping cream.

Plant type:
Shrub

Description: 3m (10ft) high by 3m (10ft) wide; small yellow flowers

Native habitat: Tropical grassland; W Africa

Parts of plant used:
Leaves, roots, fruit

Growing and harvesting

- Prefers light soil in part shade.
- Sow seed when ripe. Or transplant suckers during the tropical rainy season.
- Flowers appear after the rainy season; fruit will follow.
- Harvest leaves any time, then dry. Pick fruit when ripe, and dry. Dig up five-year-old roots in spring, and dry.

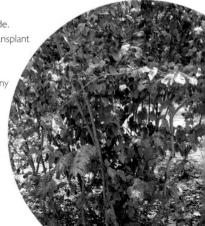

Lore and traditional uses
- In western Africa, kinkeliba is used to treat malaria and intestinal worms, as well as to aid weight loss and the body's ability to detoxify.
- West Africans use kinkeliba twigs to weave sturdy baskets.

Enhancing mind and spirit
- To encourage positive thoughts about a new beginning, take 1 cup kinkeliba leaf infusion (see first preparation, right), as necessary.

Caring for your body
- To boost energy, aid weight loss and help detoxify the blood and liver, take 1 cup kinkeliba leaf infusion (see first preparation, right) up to three times daily.
- To reduce swelling or abscesses, or speed healing of wounds, apply dried kinkeliba ointment (see second preparation, right) to the affected areas two or three times daily.
- To ease lower back pain, add 2 cups kinkeliba decoction (see third preparation, right) to a bath and soak for 20 minutes.

Core benefits
Boosts energy

Encourages weight loss

Aids detoxification

Preparations

Infusion: 1 tsp dried kinkeliba leaves in 1 cup just-boiled water. Standard method (p.20).

Ointment: Add a crushed handful dried kinkeliba fruit to olive oil to make a thin paste.

Decoction: 30g (1oz) fresh or 60g (2oz) dried kinkeliba root in 750ml (1½ pints) water. Standard method (p.20).

143

Hawthorn *Crataegus monogyna*

Research in Germany and Japan has confirmed that this familiar English hedgerow shrub supplies a potent cardiac and circulation tonic. The flowering tops (leaves and flowers) and the haws (red false fruit) treat kidney-related heart weakness, as well as thickening of the heart tissue, artery spasm and irregular heartbeat. By improving circulation in the arteries, hawthorn helps ease age-related circulation problems, such as numbness in the lower legs and poor memory and confusion (caused by reduced bloodflow to the brain). Strong antioxidants in the haws help prevent or reduce the degeneration of blood vessels.

Plant type: Hardy deciduous shrub

Description: 6m (20ft) high by 6m (20ft) wide; dense white flower clusters

Native habitat: Cool temperate; Europe, N Africa

Parts of plant used: Haws, flowering tops

Growing and harvesting

- Succeeds in all but the very poorest acid soils, but prefers a well-drained, moisture-retentive, loamy soil in full sun.
- For best results, sow seeds in a greenhouse in autumn when ripe.
- Harvest open flowers in late spring and leaves in summer, then dry. Pick haws in autumn to dry or juice.

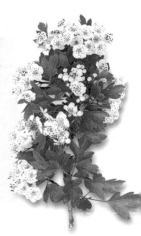

144

Lore and traditional uses

- In Greek myth, the hawthorn is associated with Hymen, the god of weddings, and was used in marriage garlands.
- During World War I, soldiers used young hawthorn leaves as a substitute for tobacco.

Enhancing mind and spirit

- To assuage extreme stress or grief, put 2 drops hawthorn flower essence (see pp.34–5) in a glass of water and sip throughout the day.

Caring for your body

- As a general heart tonic or to regulate abnormal heart rhythms, take 1 tsp hawthorn tincture (see first preparation, right) three times daily.
- To soothe the nerves after a stressful day, drink 1 or 2 cups hawthorn decoction (see second preparation, right).
- To treat boils, sores and skin ulcers, make a poultice (see p.23) of flowering hawthorn tops and apply fresh, morning and evening.

Core benefits

Supports the heart

Relaxes the nerves

Mild diuretic

Preparations

Tincture: Either 200g (7oz) dried haws or 200g (7oz) dried flowering hawthorn tops in 1 litre (2 pints) vodka-water mix. Standard method (see p.20).

Decoction: Boil 30g (1oz) dried haws in 750ml (1½ pints) water for 15 minutes only, then use the standard method (p.20).

145

Eleuthero *Eleutherococcus senticosus*

Previously called Siberian ginseng, this herb is popular with athletes as it increases stamina and improves the body's ability to recover after exertion. Regular use can restore vigour, improve memory and increase longevity, while research indicates that it may also increase sperm count in men and even kill some cancer cells. Avoid taking eleuthero for longer than three months without a two-week break.

Plant type:
Hardy, deciduous shrub

Description: 2m (7ft) high by 1.5m (5ft) wide; umbels of flowers

Native habitat: Cool temperate; E Asia, Siberia

Parts of plant used: Roots, leaves, branches

Growing and harvesting
• Prefers a moderately rich, well-drained soil and sun, but can grow in partial shade.
• Sow ripe seeds in autumn in a greenhouse. Or grow from newly matured wood cuttings.
• Harvest roots in autumn and dry.

Lore and traditional uses
• Explorers traditionally take eleuthero root to prevent stress-related illness.
• In China, eleuthero is used

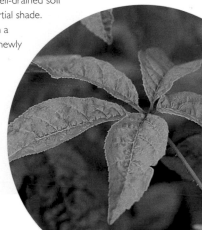

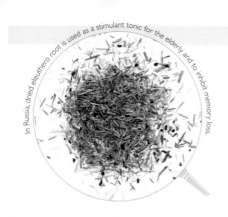

In Russia, dried eleuthero root is used as a stimulant tonic for the elderly and to inhibit memory loss.

as an energy tonic that reinforces *chi* (see p.18) and invigorates the spleen and kidneys.

Enhancing mind and spirit

- To ease grief, take 1 tsp eleuthero tincture (see first preparation, right) three times daily for up to two months.

Caring for your body

- To increase energy and endurance, take 2 or 3 size 00 capsules filled with eleuthero powder (see p.21) two or three times daily.
- To relieve stress-induced hypertension, fatigue or insomnia, drink 1 cup eleuthero decoction (see second preparation, right) up to three times daily, as necessary.

Preparations

Tincture: 200g (7oz) dried or 400g (14oz) fresh eleuthero root in 1 litre (2 pints) vodka-water mix. Standard method (p.20).

Decoction: 30g (1oz) dried or 60g (2oz) fresh eleuthero root in 750ml (1½ pints) water. Standard method (p.20).

Reishi mushroom *Ganoderma lucidum*

This long-stalked, shiny, chestnut-brown mushroom is the ultimate Taoist elixir of life. Reishi mushrooms improve circulation, lower blood pressure, are calming and pain-relieving (particularly for arthritis pain), and ease asthma, bronchitis, allergies and insomnia. The mushrooms also boost the immune system, reduce free radicals and inhibit tumours (the government in Japan recognizes reishi as an official anti-cancer treatment). As a mood-elevating substance, reishi is taken to help bring about a spiritual transformation. Consult a herbalist before taking reishi if you are pregnant or breastfeeding, or taking blood-thinning medication. Never take reishi for more than three months without a two-week break.

Growing and harvesting
- Grow reishi indoors by culturing wild reishi spores on plum-tree sawdust. You'll need to be patient – the process is complex and will take about two years.
- Harvest the mushroom when it has produced spores, but not yet released them.

Plant type:
Fungus

Description: Up to 30cm (1ft) high; long stalk, shiny, hard, fan-shaped cap

Native habitat: All temperate and tropical; worldwide

Parts of plant used:
Fruit body with mycelium (mass of thread-like, germinated spores)

Preparations

Decoction: Simmer 4½ tsp chopped fresh or dried reishi mushroom in 750ml (1½ pints) water for 10 minutes, then allow to steep for a further 30 minutes. Strain.

Tincture: 30g (1oz) dried reishi mushroom in 1 litre (2 pints) vodka-water mix. Standard method (p.20).

Lore and traditional uses

• In Taoism, reishi is the "Mushroom of Immortality", once reserved for the Chinese emperor to promote his longevity.

Enhancing mind and spirit

• To enhance spiritual receptivity, drink 1 cup reishi decoction (see first preparation, left) three times daily.

• To calm the mind and lend clarity to an otherwise muddled existence, take 1 tsp reishi tincture (see second preparation, left) three times daily.

Caring for your body

• To ease rheumatoid arthritis, take 1 tsp reishi mushroom tincture (see second preparation, left) three times daily.

• To lower blood pressure, take 2 size 00 capsules of reishi powder (see p.21) daily, as needed.

Core benefits

Boosts vitality

Antioxidant

Fights tumours

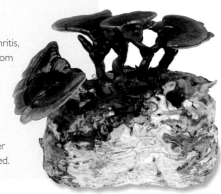

Goji berries *Lycium chinense*

The Taoist master and herbalist Li Qing Yuen reportedly lived to the staggering age of 256 – his longevity attributed partly to a daily portion of goji berries. Also known as wolfberries, they have one of the highest antioxidant contents of any food. They slow the aging process by fighting free radicals (which damage the body's cells), enhancing the immune system, fighting heart disease, and protecting the skin from sun damage. The berries have a slightly chewy texture.

Plant type: Hardy deciduous shrub

Description: 2.5m (8ft) high by 2m (7ft) wide; purple flowers

Native habitat: Cool temperate; E Asia

Parts of plant used: Fruit, root bark, leaves

Growing and harvesting
- Grows easily in well-drained soils in sun.
- Sow seeds in early spring in a greenhouse, and keep them there, protected from frost, over the first winter. Alternatively, propagate by separating suckers from a mature plant and replanting in late winter.
- Harvest berries when ripened to scarlet. Use fresh, or dry.

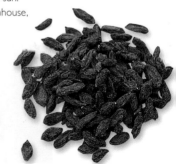

150

Lore and traditional uses

- As well as for longevity, Chinese herbalists use goji berries, root bark and, occasionally, leaves to lift the spirits and tone the liver, kidneys and blood.

Enhancing mind and spirit

- To boost your spiritual well-being take 1 cup goji berry decoction (see first preparation, right) three times daily.

Caring for your body

- To boost your intake of free-radical-fighting antioxidants, sprinkle a large handful of fresh goji berries on your breakfast cereal daily.
- To treat weakening eyesight, macular degeneration or glaucoma, drink 1 tsp goji berry tincture (see second preparation, right) three times daily.
- To strengthen the blood vessels and improve the circulation, or – for men – to boost sperm production, drink 1 cup goji berry decoction (see first preparation, right) two to three times daily.

Core benefits

Antioxidant

Improves eyesight

Strengthens circulation

Preparations

Decoction: 30g (1oz) dried or 60g (2oz) fresh goji berries in 750ml (1½ pints) water. Standard method (p.20).

Tincture: 200g (7oz) dried or 400g (14oz) fresh goji berries in 1 litre (2 pints) vodka-water mix. Standard method (p.20).

Alfalfa *Medicago sativa*

Recognized as a herbal medicine for more than 1,500 years, highly nutritious alfalfa has a leaf that is rich in antioxidants, protein, minerals and vitamins, and helps lower cholesterol, boost immunity, regulate blood sugar, relieve arthritis, restore estrogen levels, and alkalize the system (too much acidity leads to ill health). However, the leaf's high fibre content makes alfalfa difficult to use fresh except as young shoots or sprouted seeds. You can use powdered alfalfa leaves in food, as an infusion or in capsules.

Plant type: Hardy perennial legume

Description: 1m (3ft) high by 60cm (2ft) wide; deep roots

Native habitat: All temperate; SW Asia, Europe, USA

Parts of plant used: Flowers, leaves, stems, seeds

Growing and harvesting

- Succeeds in most soils in full sun.
- Use seeds inoculated with *Rhizobium* bacteria, enabling the plant to convert air nitrogen into plant nitrogen. Pre-soak seeds for 12 hours in warm water. Sow in spring *in situ*.
- After second year, harvest leaves any time, then dry. Or eat raw young, fresh shoots, or sprouted seeds.

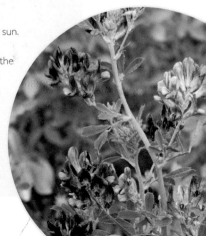

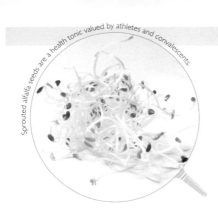

Sprouted alfalfa seeds are a health tonic valued by athletes and convalescents

Lore and traditional uses
• North American Indians used alfalfa's aerial parts to treat jaundice and stem bleeding.

Enhancing mind and spirit
• To encourage your dreams to reveal your subconscious, take 1 tsp alfalfa leaf powder in clary sage infusion (see p.273) before bed.

Caring for your body
• To enhance longevity, sprinkle 1 tsp alfalfa leaf powder on food two or three times daily.
• To ease arthritis, take 1 cup alfalfa leaf infusion (see first preparation, right) three times daily.
• To treat skin infections, apply alfalfa juice (second preparation, right) directly to the site.

Preparations

Infusion: 1 tsp dried alfalfa leaves in 1 cup just-boiled water. Standard method (p.20).

Juice: Place a handful of raw alfalfa sprouts in a blender and whiz until smooth.

Sweet cicely *Myrrhis odorata*

The botanical name of this woodland plant comes from the Greek for "perfume": the soft leaves have a myrrh-like scent with hints of moss and aniseed. The late-spring umbels of nectar-rich, white flowers give way to large, green (unripe) seeds in early summer, which have a nutty, aniseed taste and provide an aromatic furniture polish. The leaves neutralize acidity, making tart food, such as rhubarb, seem sweeter, reducing the need for sugar. A sweet cicely root infusion provides a general tonic, a digestive and a mild antiseptic; the leaves are prescribed for anemia in the elderly.

Plant type:
Hardy perennial

Description: 1m (3ft) high by 1m (3ft) wide; feathery, aniseedy leaves

Native habitat: Cool temperate; Europe

Parts of plant used:
Leaves, root, seeds

Growing and harvesting

- Prefers moist, rich soil in light shade.
- Sow seeds in late summer as soon as ripe (when they turn black). Keep moist.
- Harvest roots in autumn, then dry; pick the feathery leaves any time to use fresh.

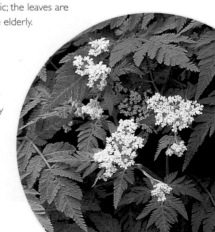

Lore and traditional uses
- In the Middle Ages, the green seeds of sweet cicely were sprinkled on salads and used to flavour liqueurs.
- Early herbalists used sweet cicely root ointment as an antiseptic to soothe wounds, relieve gout, and treat dog and snake bites.

Enhancing mind and spirit
- For a cheerful nudge toward enhancing all your senses, put 2 drops sweet cicely flower essence (see pp.34–5) in a glass of water and sip throughout the day.

Caring for your body
- To gently stimulate the stomach and reduce flatulence, take 1 cup sweet cicely leaf infusion (see first preparation, right) up to three times daily, as required.
- To reduce the build-up of uric acid in cases of gout, drink 1 cup sweet cicely decoction (see second preparation, right) three times daily, and apply a compress (see p.23) of double-strength decoction to the area.

Core benefits

Aids digestion

Cleanses urinary tract

Eases respiration

Preparations

Infusion: 2 tsp fresh sweet cicely leaves in 1 cup just-boiled water. Standard method (p.20).

Decoction: 30g (1oz) dried or 60g (2oz) fresh sweet cicely root in 750ml (1½ pints) water. Standard method (p.20). (For double-strength, use double the root in the same amount of water.)

155

Peony *Paeonia officinalis*

With voluptuous blossoms and a potent root, this herb has been used medicinally for at least 2,000 years. The European peony (*P. officinalis*), as well as the Chinese peony (*P. lactiflora*) and the tree peony (*P. suffruticosa*), is used to treat epilepsy and eczema, and as an antibacterial and a sedative. The roots of all three species contain peoniflorin, which can help reduce blood sugar, fight tumours, protect against Parkinson's disease and prevent strokes. Research in Japan found that paeoniflorin helps protect the body's cells against damage by toxins, free radicals and heat, and shows great potential for new anti-aging medicines.

Plant type:
Hardy perennial

Description: 1m (3ft) high by 60cm (2ft) wide; red, pink or white flowers

Native habitat: Cool temperate; Europe

Parts of plant used: Flowers, roots, seeds

Growing and harvesting

- Enjoys deep, alkaline—neutral soil, in sun or light shade.
- Sow ripe seeds in a cold frame. Or divide mature plants in spring or autumn.
- Harvest root from two-year-old plants, then dry; pick flowers in spring.

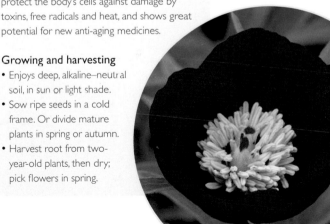

Lore and traditional uses

- In Greek myth, the moon goddess, Selene, created the peony and gave it to Pæon, physician to the Olympian gods.
- In Japan, the plant is considered the "food of dragons" and the flowers are eaten as a vegetable.

Enhancing mind and spirit

- To open the heart *chakra* (see p.17) to abundant, generous love, put 2 drops pink peony flower essence (see pp.34–5) in a glass of water and sip throughout the day.

Caring for your body

- To delay memory loss and support healthy brain function, take 1 tsp peony tincture (see first preparation, right) three times daily.
- To lower cholesterol levels, drink 1 cup peony decoction (see second preparation, right) three times daily.
- To help balance blood-sugar levels, take 2 or 3 size 00 capsules filled with powdered peony root (see p.21) daily, as needed.

Core benefits

Improves memory

Lowers cholesterol

Balances blood sugar

Preparations

Tincture: 40g (1½oz) dried peony root in 1 litre (2 pints) vodka-water mix. Standard method (p.20).

Decoction: 30g (1oz) dried peony root in 750ml (1½ pints) water. Standard method (p.20).

157

Ginseng *Panax ginseng*

The fleshy aromatic taproot of this woodland plant is a famous *yang* (see p.18) stimulant. It is the original adaptogen (see p.136), strengthening the whole body by increasing the efficiency of the endocrine, metabolic, circulatory and digestive systems. Gingseng root reduces stress by increasing numbers of oxygen-carrying red blood cells and immune-strengthening white blood cells, and by eliminating toxins. Avoid taking ginseng for more than six weeks continuously (break for two weeks, then resume if necessary).

Plant type:
Hardy perennial

Description: 80cm (2½ft) high by 60cm (2ft) wide; long stem with leaflets

Native habitat: Cool temperate; NE China, Korea

Parts of plant used: Roots

Growing and harvesting

• Prefers moist, humus-rich soil in shade.
• Sow ripe seeds; keep in greenhouse for first winter. Or separate rhizome or "neck" of older plants from roots and replant in spring.
• Harvest roots in autumn once plants are six years old. Use fresh, or dry.

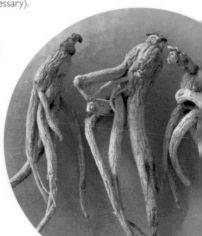

Lore and traditional uses

- Ginseng has been used therapeutically for more than 5,000 years, making it one of China's most ancient and valued herbs.
- In the 17th century, an ambassador of the King of Siam visited Louis XIV of France and gave him precious ginseng root as a gift.

Enhancing mind and spirit

- To help the body to process emotional stress, drink 1 cup ginseng decoction (see first preparation, right) up to three times daily, as needed (breaking and resuming if necessary).

Caring for your body

- To enhance physical endurance, take 2 or 3 size 00 capsules ginseng root powder (see p.21) three times daily, as required.
- To speed up recovery from a cold, take 1 tsp ginseng tincture (see second preparation, right) three times daily until you are better.
- To improve male fertility, take 2 or 3 size 00 capsules filled with ginseng root powder (see p.21) three times daily, as required.

Core benefits

Enhances body systems

Boosts immunity

Anti-aging

Preparations

Decoction: Boil 2 tsp dried or 4 tsp fresh ginseng root in 2 cups water for 10–15 minutes. Strain, then drink.

Tincture: 20g (¾oz) dried or 40g (1½oz) fresh ginseng root in 1 litre (2 pints) vodka-water mix. Standard method (p.20).

Maral root *Rhaponticum carthamoides*

Also known as leuzea, Siberian maral root
has gained the attention of body-builders as
it helps the body synthesize muscle protein,
build muscle and repair damaged muscle
tissue. It also increases endurance, reflexes and
concentration, and reduces the body's recovery
time following exertion. This tall plant has a
woody rhizome and wiry roots with a resinous
scent. In its second year, it bears flower stems
topped with a dense thistle-like cluster of violet
florets. Extensive use of the root may cause
high blood pressure. Avoid during pregnancy.

Plant type:
Hardy perennial

Description: 1.5m (5ft)
high by 45cm (1½ft) wide;
solitary violet flowers

Native habitat: Cool temperate; S Siberia, Mongolia

Parts of plant used:
Roots

Growing and harvesting
- Prefers deep, well-drained,
  moderately fertile soil in sun.
- Sow seeds (just covered with
  soil) in autumn. Or propagate
  by dividing the plant in
  spring or early autumn.
- Harvest rootstock with
  growing roots after two
  years in early autumn.
  Dry for four to six days.

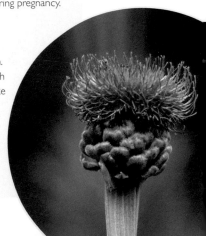

160

Lore and traditional uses

- Maral root is a Russia's "Elixir of Longevity", used to overcome fatigue and impotence.
- In Siberia, the root provides fodder to improve animals' tolerance of the cold.
- In Tibet, maral root is used in blends for lung and kidney diseases, jaundice, fever and angina.

Enhancing mind and spirit

- To help break addictive habits, take $^1/_3$ cup maral root infusion (see first preparation, right) three times daily. (Note: never take more than 1 cup infusion in total daily.)
- To aid memory, fill 60 size 00 capsules with 300g (10½oz) powdered maral root (see p.21); take 2 a day at breakfast for 30 days.

Caring for your body

- To increase physical endurance, take ½ tsp maral tincture (see second preparation, right) three times daily for 10 to 20 days.
- To treat impotence, fill size 00 capsules with 200–300g (7–10½oz) powdered maral root (see p.21) and take 2 a day for 30 days.

Core benefits

Enhances endurance

Improves memory

Builds muscle

Preparations

Infusion: Infuse 3 tsp finley chopped dried maral root in 1 cup just-boiled water for 4–5 hours, then filter. (One dosage is $^1/_3$ cup.)

Tincture: Grind 30g (1oz) dried maral root into 5–10mm (¼–½in) pieces. Stir into 150ml (¹/₃ pint) vodka. Steep for 3–5 days at room temperature, then filter.

Golden root *Rhodiola rosea*

Research in Russia has shown that golden root (or rose root) has extraordinary anti-aging properties, because it can reduce the effects of internal and external stresses on the body. It also makes us *feel* younger and more positive, because it can optimize the brain's levels of the good-mood hormones, serotonin and dopamine. Perhaps most important of all is the fact that golden root can increase DNA repair within the body's cells, rejuvenating them. Taken at lower doses, this herb has a stimulating effect on the body; at higher doses it is more sedative.

Plant type:
Hardy perennial

Description: 30cm (1ft) high by 30cm (1ft) wide; fleshy leaves; yellow flowers

Native habitat: Mountain; C Asia, N America, Europe

Parts of plant used:
Roots

Growing and harvesting

- Tolerates rocky soil; easy to grow in full sun.
- Propagate in autumn, in well-drained soil, from root pieces with a growing bud and hair roots.
- Harvest five-year-old roots in autumn; slice into strips that are 10cm (4in) long. Dry in shade; store in paper bags for up to three years.

Lore and traditional uses

- Viking legend praises golden root's powers to increase longevity and enhance strength.
- Siberian couples are given golden root to enhance fertility and produce healthy babies.
- Tibetan Sherpas chew golden root to treat altitude sickness while mountain climbing.

Enhancing mind and spirit

- To improve mental faculties, take 1 tsp golden root tincture (see first preparation, right) two or three times daily.
- To relieve depression and anxiety, take 1 cup golden root infusion (see second preparation, right) up to three times daily, as required.

Caring for your body

- To reduce cell damage and defy aging, take 1 or 2 size 00 capsules filled with powdered golden root (see p.21) three times daily.
- To reduce fatigue and promote deep, restful sleep, take 2 or 3 size 00 capsules filled with powdered golden root (see p.21) immediately before bedtime, as needed.

Core benefits

Rejuvenates cells

Improves recall

Alleviates anxiety

Preparations

Tincture: 200g (7oz) dried or 400g (14oz) fresh golden root in 1 litre (2 pints) vodka-water mix. Standard method (p.20).

Infusion: Finely chop 3 tsp dried golden root. Place the chopped root in 1 cup just-boiled water and infuse for at least 4 hours. Strain.

Sage *Salvia officinalis*

One Chinese proverb asks, "How can a man grow old with sage in his garden?" Packed with youth-giving qualities, sage has long been considered a cure-all. Its botanical name comes from the Latin *salvere*, to cure or to save. The leaves provide a well-known digestive, a nerve and blood tonic, and a mouth and throat antiseptic; the aerial parts contain hormone triggers that aid the female reproductive system. Current research is investigating sage's antioxidant and blood-sugar-balancing potential, and its use as a memory aid. Avoid large doses if you are pregnant, or if you have epilepsy.

Plant type: Hardy, evergreen shrub

Description: 60cm (2ft) high by 60cm (2ft) wide; mauve-blue flowers

Native habitat: Warm temperate; N Africa

Parts of plant used: Leaves, flowers, essential oil (from leaves)

Growing and harvesting

- Requires well-drained, light soil in a sunny position.
- Sow seeds in spring in a greenhouse. Or take cuttings in late spring, summer or autumn.
- Pick leaves fresh all year; or before flowering in midsummer to dry.

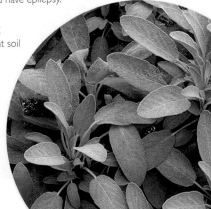

Lore and traditional uses

- In Traditional Chinese Medicine, sage is a *yin* tonic (see p.18) and supports the nerves.
- The ancient Greeks believed that with sage in the garden a family would never need to see a doctor.

Enhancing mind and spirit

- For an uplifting tonic to strengthen the nervous system, relieve anxiety and depression, improve memory and sharpen the senses, drink a small glass of sage tonic wine (see first preparation, right) every day with your evening meal.

Caring for your body

- For a sore throat, bleeding gums, loose teeth or mouth inflammations, gargle with sage leaf infusion (see second preparation, right) four to six times daily, as required.
- To reduce hot flashes during menopause, or to stem lactation when weaning, take 2 or 3 size 00 capsules of powdered sage leaves (see p.21) up to three times daily, as necessary.

Core benefits

Stimulating

Antiseptic

Balances hormones

Preparations

Tonic wine: 200g (7oz) dried or 100g (3½oz) fresh sage leaves in 1 litre (2 pints) wine. Use white wine for green sage leaves and red wine for purple. Otherwise, use standard method (p.22).

Infusion: 1 tsp dried or 2 tsp fresh sage leaves in 1 cup just-boiled water. Standard method (p.20).

Grapevine *Vitis vinifera*

The grapevine is one of the oldest continuously cultivated plants in history. The grapes provide a refreshing blood tonic, while the leaves have long been used as an astringent and anti-inflammatory to treat fragile and varicose veins. The branch sap provides an eyewash and the seeds yield a light, fine oil (used in both cooking and massage) that can reduce high blood pressure and inhibit cancer. Red grape skins contain the compound resveratrol, which protects the heart, boosts bone density, reduces colds, inhibits cataracts and, applied topically, can prevent the spread of herpes.

Plant type:
Hardy vine

Description: Up to 35m (115ft) long; large green or purple leaves

Native habitat: All temperate; C and S Europe

Parts of plant used:
Fruit, seeds, leaves, sap

Growing and harvesting
- Prefers deep, well-drained, moist soil in full or partial sun.
- Sow seeds autumn to spring. Or propagate from cuttings taken midwinter to spring.
- Harvest grapes and seeds when ripe in late summer, then crush and dry (drink the strained juice).

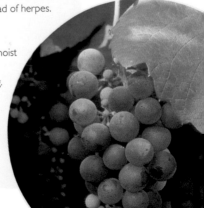

Lore and traditional uses
- Tomb texts show that Egyptians ate grapes at least 6,000 years ago.
- Several ancient Greek philosophers praised the healing power of grapes, and Hippocrates (c.460–c.375BCE) was among the first doctors to prescribe wine as a medicine.

Enhancing mind and spirit
- To ease the mind, add 1 tsp passionflower tincture (200g/7oz dried leaves; standard method, p.20) to 1 small glass red grape wine.

Caring for your body
- To boost your intake of antioxidants to fight aging, and to improve circulation, take 1 tsp grape tincture (see first preparation, right) three times daily.
- To protect against allergies, take 2 or 3 size 00 capsules filled with powdered red grape seed and skin (see p.21) three times daily.
- To treat varicose veins, apply grape seed and skin infused oil (see second preparation, right) to the affected veins two or three times daily.

Core benefits

Antioxidant

Inhibits allergies

Improves circulation

Preparations

Tincture: 200g (7oz) dried or 400g (14oz) fresh grape seeds and skins (use red grapes) in 1 litre (2 pints) vodka-water mix. Standard method (p.20).

Infused oil: Fill a bottle ¾ full with dried red grape skins and seeds. Fill to the top with olive oil, then infuse as directed on p.23.

CHAPTER 6

Cleansing Herbs

Some might say that the path to well-being begins with this chapter – the cleansing herbs are those that help rid our bodies of the accumulated pollutants that enter us via air, water, food and the products we use.

Of course, the body makes a valiant effort to combat toxicity through several in-built systems of elimination: the lungs, which enable us to breathe out toxins; lymphatic drainage; the blood and the digestive system, which filter toxins through the liver and kidneys; and the skin, which expels toxins via the pores.

However, the sheer quantity of pollutants that bombard us can overwhelm these systems and the overload can lead to chronic illnesses, such as irritable bowel or chronic fatigue syndromes. Early signs that you are in need of a detox may be tiredness, poor sleep, bad breath, sallow skin and aching joints.

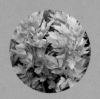 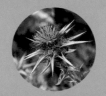

All the herbs in this chapter support the body's detox systems. For a general boost to the systems of elimination, and especially the blood, kidneys and liver, you can't beat dandelion. Milk thistle, nettle, parsley and burdock are other good liver-detoxifiers, while the kidneys also benefit from nettle, parsley and lovage. Lovage will boost the lymphatic system, too, as will hyssop, which also clears the skin and blood. There are countless permutations. Explore the chapter and find out what works for you. When your sleep and digestion improve, your skin is clear, and you feel less stressed, you've got the balance right. Also, drink lots of water during a detox to flush out toxins.

As well as taking the detox herbs using the preparations, try to include them in your diet: use dandelion or nettles in salads, and chop parsley into meat dishes or onto potatoes.

Yarrow *Achillea millefolium*

Yarrow's botanical name honours the Greek warrior Achilles, who was instructed in a dream to use yarrow leaves to staunch the blood of his soldiers' wounds. Yarrow's flowering tops yield a cleansing tonic, a digestive, and a diuretic that is used to treat high blood pressure; and a useful tonic wash for oily skin. The flowers alone may also be used to treat eczema and allergy-related catarrh. The unsung powers of this feathery herb include root secretions that intensify the medicinal actions of other herbs growing nearby. Using too much yarrow can make the skin sensitive to sunlight and cause a rash. Avoid yarrow during pregnancy.

Plant type:
Hardy perennial

Description: 1m (3ft) high by 60cm (2ft) wide; dense white flower heads

Native habitat: Cool temperate; Europe, W Asia

Parts of plant used:
Flowers, leaves, stems

Growing and harvesting

• Prefers well-drained soil in sun.

• Sow seeds in spring or early autumn in a cold frame. Alternatively, divide plants at any time of year.

• Harvest aerial parts when plant is in flower. Use fresh, or dry.

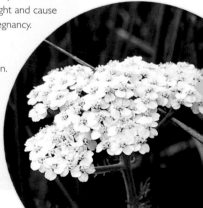

Lore and traditional uses

- The Druids used yarrow stems to divine the weather conditions, and the Chinese used them with the *I Ching* to divine the future.
- The Pennsylvania Dutch called yarrow *schoof ribba* and used the whole plant as a "sweating fever tonic" and a leaf tea to improve the action of the liver and gall bladder.

Enhancing mind and spirit

- To stimulate the meridians (see p.18) and protect and strengthen the aura, put 2 drops yarrow flower essence (see pp.34–5) in a glass of water and sip throughout the day.

Caring for your body

- To encourage a cleansing sweat after a fever, take 1 cup yarrow infusion (see first preparation, right) up to three times daily.
- To stem bleeding in a shaving cut, chew a few yarrow leaves and apply them to the wound.
- To improve the body's nutrient absorption, take 1 tbsp yarrow tonic wine (see second preparation, right) before meals, as needed.

Core benefits

Encourages sweating

Staunches blood flow

Aids digestion

Preparations

Infusion: ½ tsp dried or 1 tsp fresh yarrow flowers and/or leaves in 1 cup just-boiled water. Standard method (p.20).

Tonic wine: 80g (3oz) crushed fresh or dry yarrow flowers in 1 litre (2 pints) white wine for 30 days. Standard method (p.22).

Aloe vera *Aloe vera*

A cornerstone of Cleopatra's beauty regime, the almost tasteless clear gel inside aloe leaves offers remarkable gifts. It soothes, heals and moisturizes the skin and inhibits itching and scarring. Taken internally, it provides essential nutrients (including vitamins A, C and E), a gentle laxative, an immunity stimulant and a blood-sugar balancer. The yellow-green bitter sap in the leaf wall provides protection against UV rays and shows anti-cancer activity.

Plant type: Evergreen succulent perennial

Description: 1m (3ft) high by 60cm (2ft) wide; orange flowers; thick leaves

Native habitat: Warm temperate; N Africa

Parts of plant used: Leaf gel, leaf sap, flowers

Growing and harvesting

- Prefers well-drained soil in sun; can grow indoors, but out of direct sun.
- Grow from offsets taken from around the base. Or sow seeds in spring indoors.
- Harvest lower leaves any time: cut each leaf diagonally across its base. Stand in a jar for 10 minutes to drain sap (store this separately). Slice open leaf, scrape out gel and use immediately.

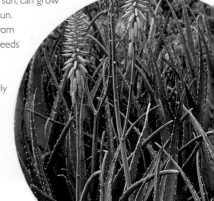

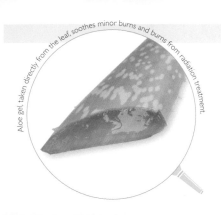

Aloe gel, taken directly from the leaf, soothes minor burns and burns from radiation treatment.

Heals the skin

Anti-inflammatory

Boosts immunity

Lore and traditional uses

• Oriental, Persian, Greek and Roman physicians all used the whole aloe vera leaf to treat ailments as diverse as tonsillitis and insomnia.

Enhancing mind and spirit

• To increase your sensitivity to others, put 2 drops aloe vera flower essence (see pp.34–5) in a glass of water; sip throughout the day.

Caring for your body

• For wounds, bedsores, eczema and minor burns, apply aloe gel (see first preparation, right) three to five times daily, until healed.

• To moisturize the skin, apply aloe gel lotion (see second preparation, right) twice daily.

Preparations

Aloe gel (direct application): Slice open a length of leaf. To apply the gel, stroke the leaf's inner surface against the areas of affected skin.

Aloe gel lotion: Cut open several leaves and scrape the gel into a pan. Simmer slowly until thickened to a desired consistency. Store in jars in the refrigerator for up to 1 month.

173

Burdock *Arctium lappa*

If you walk in the countryside and find yourself – or your dog – clothed in burrs, you have probably passed a burdock. The huge leaves and thick root of this wild herb have long been used in cleansing remedies. Herbalists value the root especially for its ability to detoxify the blood – particularly of heavy metals, such as mercury and lead – and tests show that it may provide a mild cancer inhibitor. Burdock leaf helps reduce persistent bacterial and fungal infections and re-establish a normal community of gut bacteria. Burdock is usually taken in combination with other herbs – for example, dandelion and burdock wine makes a popular digestive tonic. Avoid using burdock during pregnancy.

Growing and harvesting

- Prefers a moist, well-drained soil and partial shade.
- Sow fresh seeds, *in situ*, in autumn.
- Harvest roots of one-year-old plants in spring; use them fresh, or dry, but they contain most active ingredients when used fresh.

Plant type:
Hardy biennial

Description: 1.5m (5ft) high by 1m (3ft) wide; purple flower heads

Native habitat: Cool temperate; Europe

Parts of plant used:
Leaves, stems, roots, seeds

Preparations

Burdock syrup: Place 2 tsp ground burdock root, 1½ tsp ground dandelion root, 2.5cm (1in) fresh ginger, 2 whole star anise (crushed) and ¾ tsp citric acid in 1 litre (2 pints) water. Simmer for 30 minutes. Filter; stir in 450g (1lb) sugar. Store.

Decoction: 60g (2oz) fresh burdock root in 750ml (1½ pints) water. Standard method (p.20).

Lore and traditional uses

- Burdock is among the top 54 medicinal plants of China and is one of its longevity herbs.
- In Russia, burdock juice used to be rubbed on bald heads to stimulate hair growth.

Enhancing mind and spirit

- To encourage happy reminiscences, add 45ml (3 tbsp) burdock syrup (see first preparation, left) to 200ml (6½fl oz) iced soda water, and sip.

Caring for your body

- To clear toxins, drink 1 cup burdock decoction (see second preparation, left) up to three times daily.
- To heal persistent fungal and bacterial skin infections, including athlete's foot and acne, wash the areas twice daily with cooled burdock decoction (see second preparation, left), until cleared.

Core benefits

Purifies the blood

Cleanses the skin

Antibiotic

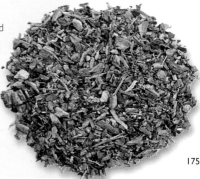

175

Hyssop *Hyssopus officinalis*

The name hyssop derives from the Hebrew word *ezob*, meaning "holy herb", and this plant was once used in rituals to purify temples and cleanse those with leprosy. Research has found that its leaves contain an antiseptic, antiviral oil and host a penicillin mould. Recent tests show that compounds in hyssop leaves can inhibit the replication of HIV-1 cells, while hyssop essential oil can help regulate blood pressure.

Growing and harvesting

- Enjoys a light, well-drained soil in a sunny position.
- Grow from seeds in spring, or from cuttings taken from spring through to autumn.
- Harvest leaves any time and flowerings tops as flowering begins. Dry, or infuse in oil.

Lore and traditional uses

- In the 1st century CE, the Romans made a hyssop wine called

Plant type: Semi-evergreen dwarf shrub

Description: 45cm (1½ft) high by 60cm (2ft) wide; blue, pink or white flowers

Native habitat: Warm temperate; Mediterranean

Part of plant used: Leaves, flowering tops, essential oil (from flowering tops)

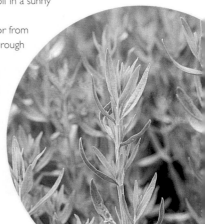

hyssopites. Knowledge of this later influenced Benedictine monks to introduce the herb to France to flavour the liqueur Chartreuse.

- In 17th-century Europe, hyssop was a popular strewing herb – the crushed leaves were scattered to mask bad odours.

Enhancing mind and spirit

- To alleviate guilt and the muscular and nervous tension that accompany it, put 4–7 drops hyssop flower essence (see pp.34–5) under the tongue, as required.
- As a general nerve tonic, drink a small glass of hyssop tonic wine (see first preparation, right) before evening meals, as required.

Caring for your body

- To reduce swelling and the colour of bruises, gently stroke infused hyssop leaf oil (see p.23) on problem areas twice daily.
- To loosen catarrh, take 1 cup hyssop leaf infusion (see second preparation, right) three times daily. To enhance the effects, sweeten with 1 tsp hyssop honey (from health stores).

Core benefits

Cleanses wounds

Expectorant

Nerve tonic

Preparations

Tonic wine: 100g (3½oz) dried or 200g (7oz) fresh hyssop leaves in 1 litre (2 pints) red wine. Standard method (p.22).

Infusion: 1 tsp dried or 3 tsp fresh hyssop leaves in 1 cup just-boiled water. Standard method (p.20).

177

Lovage *Levisticum officinale*

Lovage is a tall, handsome plant with savoury-scented leaves that make perfect additions to soups and stews. An infusion of seeds, leaves or roots reduces water retention and assists the elimination of toxins, making this a slimming, deodorizing herb. Detoxifying properties combined with antimicrobial properties make the herb useful for urinary tract problems. Lovage offers a warming tonic for the digestive and respiratory systems, easing indigestion, wind and bronchitis. Avoid lovage if you are pregnant or have kidney problems. Applied topically, it may cause a skin reaction.

Growing and harvesting

- Likes a rich, moist but well-drained soil in sun.
- Sow seeds in spring or autumn in a greenhouse, then plant in a permanent position in summer. Or propagate by dividing mature plants in spring or autumn.
- Harvest leaves before the plant flowers, and dry; pick seeds when ripe in late summer, then dry. Dig up roots of three-year-old plants in early spring or autumn. Use fresh, or dry.

Plant type:
Hardy perennial

Description: 2m (7ft) high by 1m (3ft) wide; umbels of yellowy flowers

Native habitat: Cool temperate; E Mediterranean

Parts of plant used:
Leaves, stem, root, seed leaves, essential oil (from leaves and roots)

Preparations

Infusion: 1 tsp dried or 2 tsp fresh lovage leaves in 1 cup just-boiled water. Standard method (p.20).

Cough potion: Mix 3 tsp dried lovage root, 3 tsp dried sage leaves, and 20g (¾oz) fennel seeds in 2 cups red wine. Steep for 2 days, then strain. Bottle, then store for up to 6 months.

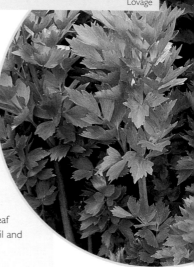

Lore and traditional uses

- In the Middle Ages, lovage root was grated raw into salads, or powdered as a condiment.
- Lovage seeds have a masculine scent that is traditionally used in perfumery.

Enhancing mind and spirit

- For an uplifting yet grounding experience, blend 2 drops lovage leaf essential oil with 1 tsp grapeseed oil and massage into the legs.

Caring for your body

- To aid slimming with a mild detoxification, take 1 cup lovage leaf infusion (see first preparation, left) three times daily, as needed.
- To aid digestion after a meal, nibble a mixture of 1 tsp each lovage, fennel, dill and coriander seeds.
- To reduce a chronic cough, take a small glass of warm lovage cough potion (see second preparation, left) after a meal, as necessary.

Core benefits
Diuretic
Aids digestion
Decongestant

179

Parsley *Petroselinum crispum*

The old English description of parsley as "the summation of all things green" aptly conjures up this fresh-tasting herb. It is a treasure chest of vitamins, minerals and chlorophyll, a substance with antiseptic, deodorizing and detoxifying properties. All parts of parsley scavenge free radicals and inhibit the release of histamine, respectively protecting the body's cells and reducing allergic reactions. Parsley relieves rheumatism, aids digestion and tones the uterine muscles. The leaf also helps condition hair and moisturize dry skin.

Plant type:
Hardy biennial

Description: 60cm (2ft) high by 60cm (2ft) wide, dense leaflets; pale flowers

Native habitat: All temperate; S Europe

Parts of plant used:
Leaves, stems, roots, seeds

Growing and harvesting

- Prefers a moist, well-drained soil in sun or partial shade.
- Three sowings of seeds can give a year-round supply of leaves. First, sow in a greenhouse in late winter. Plant out in spring. Second, sow outdoors *in situ* in midspring. Third, sow *in situ* outdoors in midsummer.

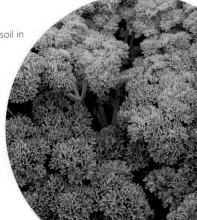

• Harvest leaves regularly to encourage fresh growth. Use fresh, or chop and then freeze (use as though fresh in preparations). Dig up root in second year. Use fresh, or dry.

Lore and traditional uses

• The ancient Greeks used parsley medicinally but did not eat it, as it was said to have grown from the blood of Archemorus, who was the harbinger of death.

Enhancing mind and spirit

• To keep the spirit feeling clear, fresh and light, nibble chopped parsley throughout the day.

Caring for your body

• To improve digestion, take 1 cup parsley leaf infusion (see first preparation, right) up to three times daily, as necessary.

• To heal bruises, sprains and insect bites, apply a poultice (see p.23) of parsley leaf or root.

• To cleanse the face, have a parsley-infused facial steam (see second preparation, right). Rest there, breathing slowly, for 10 minutes.

Core benefits
Diuretic
Freshens breath
Improves digestion

Preparations

Infusion: 1–2 tsp fresh parsley leaves in 1 cup just-boiled water. Standard method (p.20).

Facial steam: Place 2 handfuls fresh parsley leaves in a bowl and cover with 1.5 litres (3 pints) just-boiled water. To use, lean over the bowl and cover your head and the bowl with a towel (see pp.24–5).

181

Senna *Senna alexandrina*

For more than 3,500 years, from ancient Egypt to the modern day, senna has provided our bodies with a useful purgative. The leaves and pods cleanse and stimulate the lower digestive tract, and the pods alone are used as a laxative to treat constipation. The *sennoside* in the herb irritates the bowel lining, causing the muscles to contract strongly, while other active ingredients prevent fluid being absorbed out of the bowel, helping to keep the stool soft. Avoid taking senna if you have inflamed or irritated bowels, or are pregnant or breastfeeding.

Plant type:
Perennial shrub

Description: 1m (3ft) high by 1m (3ft) wide; yellow flowers

Native habitat: Warm temperate; N Africa, Mexico

Parts of plant used:
Leaves, fruit pods, flowers

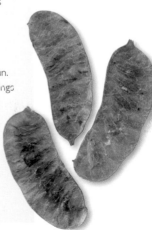

Growing and harvesting
- Requires deep, well-drained soil in full sun.
- Grow from seeds in spring or from cuttings in early summer in a greenhouse.
- Collect leaves before or during flowering, and dry; collect pods when ripe in autumn, then dry.

Lore and traditional uses
- In Ayurvedic medicine, senna is used to treat constipation, but also to treat skin

problems, jaundice, bronchitis, typhoid fever, and anemia.

- North Africans take this herb to expel intestinal worms.
- In tropical Asia, the bark of the senna shrub is used to tan leather.

Enhancing mind and spirit

- To cleanse the mind of unnecessary guilt or excessive self-judgment, and to cultivate self-compassion, put 2 drops senna flower essence (see pp.34–5) under the tongue.

Caring for your body

- As a strong treatment for constipation, take 1 cup senna laxative formula (see first preparation, right), morning and evening, for a maximum of two weeks.
- As a gentle laxative, take 1 cup senna infusion (see second preparation, right) morning and evening for up to two weeks.
- To treat ringworm and acne, apply a senna leaf poultice (see p.23) to the affected area as often as possible, until the skin has healed.

Core benefits

Strong laxative

Cleanses the colon

Treats ringworm

Preparations

Laxative formula: Mix together ½ tsp dried senna pods, ½ tsp dried licorice root powder and ½ tsp dried calendula petals. Infuse the mixture in 1 cup just-boiled water for 5–10 minutes. Strain, then drink.

Infusion: ¼–½ tsp dried senna flowers or leaves in 1 cup just-boiled water. Standard method (p.20).

183

Milk thistle *Silybum marianum*

Around 2,000 years ago, the Roman naturalist Pliny first recorded milk thistle's amazing liver-restoring properties. The plant's seeds contain the active ingredient silymarin, which alters the surface of liver cells to prevent many poisons from entering, neutralizes those that do get through, and boosts liver-cell regeneration. Remarkable milk thistle has been shown to reduce liver damage caused by alcohol, drugs, hepatitis, heavy metals and pesticides.

Plant type:
Hardy biennial

Description: 1.5m (5ft) high by 1m (3ft) wide; purple thistle flowers

Native habitat: Cool temperate; SW Europe

Parts of plant used: Leaves, seeds

Growing and harvesting
- Enjoys a well-drained, fertile soil in sun.
- Easily grown from ripe seed in summer. Alternatively, sow in spring *in situ*.
- Collect seeds when ripe, then dry.

Lore and traditional uses
- Once called the "Venus thistle", after the Roman goddess of love, this herb has also been dedicated to her Norse equivalent, Freya.

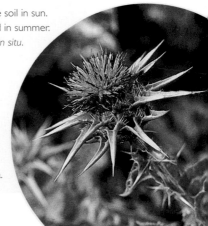

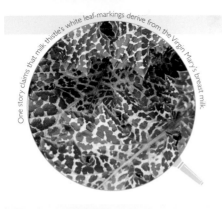

One story claims that milk thistle's white leaf-markings derive from the Virgin Mary's breast milk

Core benefits

Improves liver function

Aids digestion

Stimulates milkflow

Enhancing mind and spirit

• To accelerate your thinking, soak milk thistle seeds in water overnight. In the morning drain the seeds, chew them well, then swallow.

Caring for your body

• To strengthen the liver, aiding detoxification, take 1 200mg capsule of standardized milk thistle extract (see first preparation, right) three times daily for as long as necessary.

• To improve digestion by increasing bile, take 2 or 3 size 00 capsules filled with powdered milk thistle seed (see p.21) three times daily.

• To stimulate milkflow when breastfeeding, take 1 cup milk thistle decoction (see second preparation, right) three times daily.

Preparations

Standardized extract: As silymarin is not water-soluble, only commercial milk thistle extract will ensure that adequate amounts reach the liver. Seek advice from a herbal practitioner on a good brand.

Decoction: Simmer 1 tsp ground milk thistle seeds in 2 cups water for 10–15 minutes. Strain, then drink.

Dandelion *Taraxacum officinale*

The leaves of this golden-flowered weed are rich in vitamins A, B, C and D, as well as potassium, zinc, iron and calcium. The leaf infusion purifies the blood to help clear acne and eczema, and the milky stem latex is a mosquito repellent and helps heal warts. Dandelion root encourages the liver and gall bladder to eliminate waste, and then stimulates the kidneys to expel it via the urine. Unlike pharmaceutical diuretics, dandelion root does not deplete the body's potassium (which helps control fluid balance) – rather, it replaces it.

Plant type:
Hardy perennial

Description: 30cm (1ft) high by 20cm (8in) wide; yellow flowers; sturdy root

Native habitat: Cool temperate; Europe, N America

Part of plant used:
Flowers, leaves, stem latex, roots

Growing and harvesting
- Enjoys a rich, well-drained soil in full sun.
- Surface-sow seeds in spring. Or divide mature plants in early spring.
- Pick young, fresh leaves and flowers any time; collect leaves to dry when in flower. Dig roots in second autumn. Use fresh, or dry.

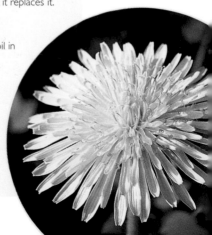

Lore and traditional uses

- Native North Americans used dandelion to treat kidney disease and skin problems.
- In England, dandelion was once called "witch gowan", which may relate to the belief that dandelions picked on Midsummer's Eve can repel witches.

Enhancing mind and spirit

- To relax the muscles and attain an easy, confident appearance, add 4 drops dandelion flower essence (see pp.34–5) to your bath.

Caring for your body

- To flush accumulated waste from the liver and gall bladder, take 1–2 tsp dandelion tincture (see first preparation, right) up to three times daily, as needed.
- To reduce acne and eczema, take 1 cup dandelion leaf infusion (see second preparation, right) three times daily.
- To purify the complexion, juice 1 dandelion root with the bases of a handful of dandelion leaves and apply as a paste to the face.

Core benefits

Diuretic

Stimulates the liver

Cleanses the skin

Preparations

Tincture: 15g (½oz) dried dandelion root powder or 30g (1oz) chopped, fresh dandelion root in 1 litre (2 pints) vodka-water mix. Standard method (p.20).

Infusion: Infuse ½–1 tsp dried or 1–2 tsp fresh dandelion leaves in 1 cup just-boiled water for 5–10 minutes. Strain, then drink.

Red clover *Trifolium pratense*

The flower of the red clover is an excellent blood-purifier, helping to improve skin conditions, boost liver health and ease arthritis. Since the 1930s, red clover flowers have become a popular treatment for breast and ovarian cancers – they contain biochanin, which fights cancer cells. The herb's antimicrobial properties are effective against tuberculosis. In Australia, the herb's estrogen-like effects on the body have led herbal-medicine manufacturers to use it to make a natural supplement that helps regulate hormone imbalances in women (such as during the menopause). Growing clover in your garden will help fertilize your soil with nitrogen.

Plant type:
Hardy perennial

Description: 30cm (1ft) high by 15cm (6in) wide; fragrant pink flowers

Native habitat: Cool temperate; Europe

Parts of plant used: Flowers, leaves, stems, roots

Growing and harvesting

• Prefers a light, well-drained soil in full sun.

• Pre-soak the seeds for 12 hours in warm water, then sow in spring *in situ*.

• Harvest flowers as they open; dry to store.

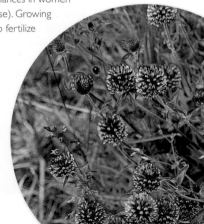

Lore and traditional uses

- Red clover is the national flower of Denmark.
- In the 19th century, herbalists used clover to treat coughs and bronchitis.

Enhancing mind and spirit

- To maintain a calm and balanced centre, easing the transition to higher awareness, put 4 drops red clover flower essence (see pp.34–5) under the tongue.

Caring for your body

- To purify the lymph and blood, and fortify the system if you suffer from cancer, drink 3 cups healing clover blend (see preparation, right) daily, for up to three months.
- To relieve eczema or psoriasis, take 3 or 4 size 00 capsules filled with powdered red clover flowers (see p.21) three times daily, for as long as necessary.
- To reduce menopausal hot flashes and night sweats, take 2 or 3 size 00 capsules filled with powdered red clover flowers (see p.21) up to three times daily, as needed.

Core benefits

Purifies the blood

Heals skin conditions

Eases menopause

Preparation

Healing clover blend: Chop and mix the following herbs (fresh or dried): 90g (3oz) red clover flowers, 90g (3oz) wood sorrel flowers, 90g (3oz) burdock root, 30g (1oz) kelp, 30g (1oz) slippery elm bark and 30g (1oz) blessed thistle head. Put 1 tsp of the blended herbs in a pan, cover with 1 cup water and boil for 5 minutes. Strain, then drink.

Stinging nettle *Urtica dioica*

Taken therapeutically, nettle's energizing leaves stimulate the bladder and kidneys to ensure rapid removal of accumulated toxins. The leaves boost circulation and clear uric acid, which relieves gout, arthritis and eczema. Young leaves, rich in vitamins, iron, zinc and chlorophyll, may be cooked as greens, brewed for beer or infused to treat anemia. Research indicates that nettle can reduce inflammation of the prostate gland and may help reduce progressive baldness in men. Heating or drying nettle leaves removes their stings, which appear only when the herb is *not* in flower.

Growing and harvesting

- Prefers a nitrogen-rich soil in part shade.
- Sow seeds in spring, just covering with soil. Or divide plants any time, and replant.
- Harvest leaves for medicinal purposes in early summer as the plant comes into flower (for culinary use, at any time); use fresh, or dry. Pick flowers in late summer and (after first year) roots in autumn. Use fresh, or dry.

Plant type:
Hardy perennial

Description: 1.5m (5ft) high by 70cm (8in) wide; irritant hairs ("stings")

Native habitat. Cool temperate; Europe, N America

Parts of plant used:
Flowers, leaves, stems, roots, fruit, seeds

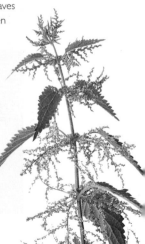

Lore and traditional uses

• Evidence in Denmark suggests that during the Bronze Age (around 4,000 years ago) nettle fibres were used to make burial shrouds.

• Egyptian papyri illustrate the use of nettle infusion to relieve arthritis and lumbago.

Enhancing mind and spirit

• To transform feelings of powerlessness, put 2 drops stinging nettle flower essence (see pp.34–5) on each wrist, as needed.

Caring for your body

• As a cleansing body tonic, take 2 cups stinging nettle leaf infusion (see first preparation, right) daily, as required.

• To ease gout, arthritis and rheumatism, drink 1 cup stinging nettle decoction (see second preparation, right) up to three times daily, for as long as necessary.

• To reduce a benign swollen prostate, take 2 or 3 size 00 capsules filled with stinging nettle root powder (see p.21) three times daily, until the swelling subsides.

Core benefits

Diuretic

Supports the prostate

Enriches the blood

Preparations

Infusion: 1 tsp dried or 2 tsp fresh stinging nettle leaves in 1 cup just-boiled water. Standard method (p.20).

Decoction: 30g (1oz) dried or 60g (2oz) fresh stinging nettle roots in 750ml (1½ pints) water. Standard method (p.20).

191

CHAPTER 7

Relaxing Herbs

Who among us, after a stressful day, doesn't long to get home, put up our feet and just relax? And who doesn't have 101 things interrupting this pleasant plan? So, with time in short supply, let nature's stress-busters take the burden.

An instant way to unwind when you get home is to sit among your herbs – even if that's just a seat by a window box filled with your precious plants. Stroke the leaves and inhale the perfumes and you will feel your cells sigh in blissful relief. As you enjoy borage, lemon balm or cowslip, pick a few leaves or flowers, then make an infusion. All three teas will alleviate headaches and nervous exhaustion.

The working day can also create muscle tension, especially if you've been sitting at a desk. In this chapter, infusions such as those of German chamomile and lime (linden) blossom can have a gentle, soothing effect on both

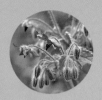 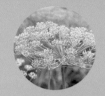 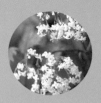

stressed muscles and nerves, helping you relax physically, as well as mentally.

For a more powerful herbal sedative, choose a herb such as valerian, which can reduce anxiety and aggression, or blue skullcap, which can deliver speedy relief from stress.

If you feel sad, or even if you suffer from mild depression, try St John's wort, renowned for its stress-relieving activity and now the number-one antidepressant in Germany.

However, the herbs in this chapter aren't only for rescuing your spirit when it's in trouble. Even without stress, the relaxing herbs offer an opportunity – an excuse, even – to indulge yourself. For a soothing, cosseted feeling, linger in a warm bath infused with a few drops of German chamomile essential oil. To envelop yourself in restorative sleep, take passionflower, dill or wild-oat tea and sleep in sheets that smell of lavender.

Dill *Anethum graveolens*

The sweet, aromatic flavour of dill is unique – it is sharpest in the seeds, weakest in the feathery leaves, and perfect in the flowering heads. The name dill, from the Norse *dylla*, means to lull or soothe, and this herb soothes digestion, stomach pains and hiccups, reduces flatulence, and lulls you to sleep. The essential oil is used in drinks, food and infant gripe water.

Plant type:
Annual

Description: 60cm (2ft) high by 20cm (8in) wide; umbels of yellow flowers

Native habitat: Warm temperate; SW Europe

Parts of plant used: Flowers, leaves, seeds, stems, fruit, essential oil (from whole plant)

Growing and harvesting
- Prefers a rich, moist, well-drained soil in sun.
- Sow seeds in spring ½cm (¼in) deep, then space seedlings out to 30cm (1ft) apart. (Don't grow dill near fennel, as doing so would muddle the flavours.)
- Pick seeds when ripe (beige); dry.

Lore and traditional uses
- An Egyptian papyrus from 1500BCE records dill as part of a painkilling recipe.
- The ancient Greeks covered their eyes with dill leaves to induce sleep.

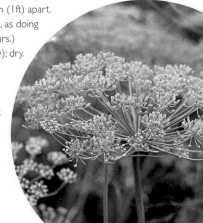

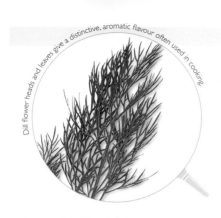

Dill flower heads and leaves give a distinctive, aromatic flavour often used in cooking.

Core benefits

Nerve tonic

Reduces stress

Aids digestion

Enhancing mind and spirit

- To expand your perspective for better self-understanding, put 2 drops dill flower essence (see pp.34–5) under the tongue.

Caring for your body

- To ease restlessness and stress accompanied by difficulty in sleeping, take 1 cup dill seed infusion (see first preparation, right) up to three times daily, as needed.

- To reduce stomach pains or flatulence, take 1 tsp dill tincture (see second preparation, right) up to three times daily, as needed.

- To relieve a colicky baby, give 1 tsp half-strength dill seed infusion (see first preparation, right), as needed.

Preparations

Infusion: 1–2 tsp slightly crushed, dried dill seeds in 1 cup just-boiled water. Standard method (p.20). (For half strength, use ½–1 tsp slightly crushed seeds in the same amount of water.)

Tincture: 200g (7oz) dried dill seeds in 1 litre (2 pints) vodka-water mix. Standard method (p.20).

Wild oats *Avena sativa*

Rich in vitamin E, minerals and protein, wild oats are a food tonic for the heart, nerves and thymus gland. The whole plant is used at the green stage (called "oat herb") to offer a soothing, restorative treatment for an exhausted nervous system. It also relieves insomnia, estrogen deficiency, depression, persistent colds and fatigue. The juice of green oats cleanses the system of uric acid, which can cause gout. The ripe plant (called "oat straw") is more useful for the skin, hair and nails.

Plant type:
Hardy annual

Description: 1m (3ft) tall; cereal plant with bladelike leaves; panicles of florets

Native habitat: Cool temperate; W Europe

Parts of plant used:
Leaves, stems, "green tops", seeds

Growing and harvesting
• Easy to grow in fertile soil in full sun.
• Sow seeds *in situ* in early spring.
• Harvest oat herb while green, before seed is hard; oat straw in autumn; and "green tops" as available.

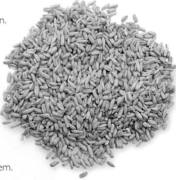

Lore and traditional uses
• The Romans considered oats a horse food and derided the "oat-eating barbarians" who toppled them.

- In Traditional Chinese Medicine, the whole oat plant is used for *chi* (see p.18) deficiency, as a nerve resorative and to lift depression.

Enhancing mind and spirit

- To help choose a new direction, take 2 drops of wild oat flower essence (use the plant's "green tops"; see pp.34–5) under the tongue.

Caring for your body

- To restore an exhausted nervous system, drink 1 cup wild oat decoction (see first preparation, right), as needed during the day.
- To soothe dry, itchy skin, such as eczema, take an oat straw bath (see second preparation, right) and drink 1 cup wild oat decoction (first preparation, right) three times daily.

Special tip

For a healthy start to the day, try my luxury porridge. Mix ½ cup oats, ½ cup milk, 1 cup water, 2 tbsp raisins, 1 mashed banana, and sprinklings of nutmeg, cinnamon and salt in a pan over a low heat. Simmer for 4 minutes.

Core benefits

Relieves insomnia

Energizes

Soothes skin conditions

Preparations

Decoction: Boil 1 tsp dried or 2 tsp fresh oat herb in 1½ cups water for 5–10 minutes. Strain, then drink immediately.

Oat straw bath: Simmer 100g (3½oz) chopped oat straw in 3 litres (6 pints) water for 20 minutes. Then add the mixture to your bath water.

Borage *Borago officinalis*

Beautiful blue-flowered borage is a herb to comfort the heart, dispel melancholy and strengthen resolve. The leaves and flowers stimulate the release of adrenaline (epinephrine), the "courage" hormone that gears the body for action under stress. Borage seed oil contains gammalinolenic acid (GLA), which eases menopausal symptoms, irritable bowel problems, eczema, bloodflow, arthritis and hangovers. Eat the leaves in moderation.

Plant type:
Hardy annual

Description: 60cm (2ft) high by 30cm (1ft) wide; blue flowers

Native habitat: All temperate; Europe

Parts of plant used: Flowers, leaves, stems, seeds

Growing and harvesting

- Grows easily in most soils in dry sun.
- Sow seeds in spring *in situ*. Or plant seedlings in late autumn – they will live over winter and get a head start in the growing season.
- Harvest leaves from late spring onward, and flowers through summer and autumn. Use herb parts fresh, or dry; store only for up to 1 year (their potency diminishes over time).

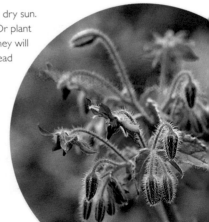

Lore and traditional uses

- According to the Roman historian Pliny, the ancient Romans used borage flowers to lighten the spirits and raise confidence.
- For courage, crusaders drank "stirrup cups" containing borage flowers and leaves as they embarked upon their lengthy voyages.

Enhancing mind and spirit

- To relieve the mind during times of stress, depression and insomnia, take 1 cup borage infusion (see first preparation, right) up to three times daily, as needed.

Caring for your body

- To ease a dry cough, or relieve a cold, fever or other signs of respiratory congestion, take 1–2 tsp borage cough syrup (see second preparation, right) three times daily, until the symptoms have passed.
- To soothe dry, irritated skin, as with acne, eczema or psoriasis, juice a handful of borage leaves, dilute the juice 50:50 with water, and apply the wash to the affected areas.

Core benefits

Uplifts the spirit

Eases coughs and colds

Calms skin conditions

Preparations

Infusion: 1 tsp dried or 2 tsp fresh borage (whole herb/any part of the herb) in 1 cup just-boiled water. Standard method (p.20).

Cough syrup: Make 2 cups (500ml/1 pint) borage infusion (see above) and mix with 2–4 tsp honey or raw sugar until the mixture turns syrupy. Refrigerate for up to 1 week.

199

St John's wort *Hypericum perforatum*

If you hold a leaf from St John's wort up to the light, you'll see what appear to be small holes. These are actually transparent cells, which contain many of the plant's active ingredients, and they give the herb its variety name *perforatum*. St John's wort is a well-known antidepressant for cases of mild depression; but, in addition, an extract of the flowers is antiviral and sedative, relieves nerve pain and reduces inflammation. You can apply the herb topically to relieve cuts, bruises and sore muscles. St John's wort may cause skin irritation if you take it internally and then go out in the sun.

Plant type:
Hardy perennial

Description: 1m (3ft) high by 45cm (1½ft) wide; yellow flowers

Native habitat: Cool temperate; Europe, C China

Parts of plant used:
Flowers, leaves, stems, fruit

Growing and harvesting

- Grows easily in well drained soil and sun.
- Sow seeds in a greenhouse when ripe, in autumn or spring. Plant out in summer.
- Harvest flowers in early summer. Use fresh, or dry.

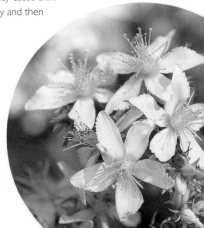

Lore and traditional uses

- The herb was named for John the Baptist and picked in full bloom on St John's Day, June 24.
- The Greek physician Hippocrates suggested taking St John's wort for "nervous unrest".

Enhancing mind and spirit

- To relieve mild to moderate depression, take 1 tsp St John's wort tincture (see first preparation, right) three times daily, for four to six months.
- To ease anxiety, take 1 cup St John's wort flower infusion (see second preparation, right) up to three times daily, as needed.

Caring for your body

- To soothe sore muscles or sprains, or to speed up the healing of bruises, wounds and infections, apply a few drops St John's wort flower-infused oil (see p.23, but steep for two months before using) to the affected area.
- To help the body fight a virus, take 1 tsp St John's wort tincture (see first preparation, right) four times daily, as needed.

Core benefits

Relieves depression

Eases sore muscles

Antiviral

Preparations

Tincture: 200g (7oz) dried or 400g (14oz) fresh St John's wort flowers in 1 litre (2 pints) vodka-water mix. Standard method (p.20).

Infusion: 1–2 tsp dried or 2 tsp fresh St John's wort flowers in 1 cup just-boiled water. Standard method (p.20).

Lavender *Lavandula angustifolia*

Although lavender had long been used to mask household smells, its value as a medicine was popularized only in the 15th century, when French glove-makers used lavender oil to scent leather – and also escaped the plague. Today, lavender infusion soothes nervous exhaustion and tension headaches, while lavender flower water can speed up cell renewal in the skin and provides an antiseptic skin wash for acne.

Growing and harvesting
- Prefers light, dry, well-drained soil in sun.
- Surface-sow seeds in a greenhouse. Keep there for the first winter, then transfer outdoors if desired. Alternatively, take 8cm (3in) cuttings in midsummer. Keep them in a greenhouse in winter.
- Cut flower stems when mostly open. Use fresh, or dry.

Lore and traditional uses
- Named from the Latin *lavare* ("to wash"), lavender was the favoured bath scent of the ancient Romans and Greeks.

Plant type:
Hardy perennial

Description: 80cm (2½ft) high by 80cm (2½ft) wide; purple or blue flowers

Native habitat: Warm temperate; Mediterranean

Parts of plant used:
Flowers, leaves, stems, essential oil (from flowers, leaves and stems)

Preparations

Infusion: 1 tsp dried or 2 tsp fresh lavender flowers in 1 cup just-boiled water. Standard method (p.20). (For triple strength, use 3 tsp dried or 6 tsp fresh flowers in 1 cup water.)

Massage blend: Mix 5 drops lavender, 2 drops fennel and 2 drops ginger essential oils in 4 tsp carrier oil, such as sweet almond oil.

- In 1150, German herbalist Hildegard of Bingen used lavender tincture to treat migraine headaches.

Enhancing mind and spirit

- To balance the emotions and induce peaceful sleep, put 1 drop lavender essential oil on each index finger and touch your temples, wrists, ankles, solar plexus, and under your nose.
- To soothe restlessness, take 1 cup lavender flower infusion (see first preparation, left) up to three times daily, as needed.

Caring for your body

- For a cell-renewing, antiseptic skin tonic, wash with triple-strength, cooled lavender flower infusion (see first preparation, left).
- To disperse cellulite, prevent fluid retention or ease muscular aches, massage the affected areas with a lavender essential oil massage blend (see second preparation, left).

Core benefits

Deeply relaxing

Soothes the mind

Tones the skin

203

German chamomile *Matricaria recutita*

The stress-reducing effects of German chamomile are legendary, but this herb is much more than just a soother. Its azulene content helps regenerate liver cells and provides an antihistamine (helping to reduce allergic reactions). An infusion of the flowers will not only help calm nervous stress, but also ease digestive problems and, applied externally, provide a refreshing skin tonic. The therapeutic properties of the other chamomile (Roman; *Chamaemeleum nobile*) are almost identical to German, but Roman chamomile has anti-tumour effects, too.

Plant type:
Hardy annual

Description: 45cm (1½ft) high by 30cm (1ft) wide; daisy flowers

Native habitat: All temperate; Europe, W Asia, India

Parts of plant used:
Flowers, leaves, essential oil (from flower heads)

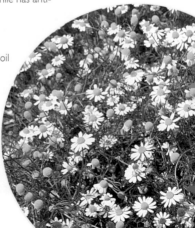

Growing and harvesting
- Grows easily in well-drained soil and sun.
- Sow seeds *in situ* in spring.
- Harvest flowers when open in summer, then dry.

Lore and traditional uses
- The ancient Egyptians dedicated chamomile to the

sun and worshipped its healing powers; they inhaled powdered chamomile flowers as snuff.
- Early European herbalists prescribed chamomile to relieve asthma and insomnia.

Enhancing mind and spirit
- To calm nervousness accompanied by muscle tension, take 1 cup German chamomile flower infusion (see first preparation, right) up to three times daily, as needed.

Caring for your body
- To stop hayfever symptoms in their tracks, put 1 drop German chamomile essential oil in each nostril, and inhale. Repeat as needed.
- To soothe sunburn or wind-chapped skin, add 1 litre (2 pints) German chamomile flower infusion (see first preparation, right) to your bath and soak in it for 20 minutes.
- To soothe indigestion, gastritis and ulcers caused by nervous anxiety, take 1 tsp German chamomile tincture (see second prepration, right) up to three times daily, as necessary.

Core benefits

Reduces anxiety

Aids digestion

Treats skin problems

Preparations

Infusion: 1 tsp dried or 2 tsp fresh German chamomile flowers in 1 cup just-boiled water. Standard method (p.20).

Tincture: 200g (7oz) dried or 400g (14oz) fresh German chamomile flowers in 1 litre (2 pints) vodka-water mix. Standard method (p.20).

205

Lemon balm *Melissa officinalis*

The 15th-century Swiss physician Paracelsus called lemon-scented lemon balm an "Elixir of Life", believing it to be one of nature's cure-alls. The herb has a long tradition as a tonic remedy that raises the spirits. Science now teaches us that it can improve memory, provide antiviral compounds to fight infection and help clean and heal wounds. The plant's refreshing, antidepressant essential oil (usually called melissa, from lemon balm's botanical name) also helps some eczema and allergy sufferers through its effects as an antihistamine.

Growing and harvesting

- Prefers a light, dry, well-drained soil in sun.
- Sow seeds *in situ*; or propagate by dividing plants in spring.
- Best used fresh, in which case harvest leaves any time. To dry, harvest before flowering – the active ingredients will remain after drying, but the leaves will lose their lemon scent. Picking stem tips to use fresh (for example, in a fresh infusion) will encourage the growing plant to sprout more leaves.

Plant type:
Hardy perennial

Description: 1m (3ft) high by 1m (3ft) wide; tiny two-lipped flowers

Native habitat: All temperate; S Europe

Parts of plant used:
Flowers, leaves, stems, essential oil (from aerial parts)

Preparations

Infusion: 1 tsp dried or 2 tsp fresh lemon balm leaves in 1 cup just-boiled water. Standard method (p.20).

Tincture: 200g (7oz) dried or 400g (14oz) fresh lemon balm leaves in 1 litre (2 pints) vodka-water mix. Standard method (p.20).

Lore and traditional uses

- Beekeepers traditionally use lemon balm to attract bees to empty hives.

Enhancing mind and spirit

- For a buoyant start to the day, replace your regular morning tea with 1 cup lemon balm leaf infusion (see first preparation, left).
- To relieve nervous tension, anxiety or depression, take 1 cup lemon balm leaf infusion (see first preparation, left) up to three times daily, for as long as necessary.

Caring for your body

- To ease stress-related high blood pressure or palpitations, take 1 tsp lemon balm tincture (see second preparation, left) three times daily, until your sense of calm returns.
- To improve your appetite or digestion, or to reduce the queasiness of a nervous stomach, take 1 tsp lemon balm tincture (see second preparation, left) up to three times daily.

Core benefits

Relieves stress

Regulates the heart

Settles the stomach

Catnip *Nepeta cataria*

The botanical name *Nepeta* derives from the Roman town of Nepeti, where catnip was once cultivated and highly valued as a seasoning and a relaxing medicinal herb. The scent of the leaf and root is well known to intoxicate cats, but it also repels rats and flea beetles (which may attack crops). The dried leaves were once smoked to relieve anxiety and stress; the leaves and flowering tops are used today to treat colds, calm upset stomachs, reduce fevers, and soothe headaches and scalp irritations. Their mild, sedative action soothes babies with colic. Avoid catnip during pregnancy.

Plant type:
Hardy perennial

Description: 1m (3ft) high by 60cm (2ft) wide; white-speckled flowers

Native habitat: Cool temperate; Europe, C Asia

Parts of plant used:
Flowers, leaves, stems, roots

Growing and harvesting

- Enjoys a light, dry soil and sun.
- Sow ripe seeds in autumn in a cold frame. Or divide mature plants in spring or autumn; or take cuttings in early summer.
- Pick flowering tops in late summer; leaves any time. Use fresh, or dry.

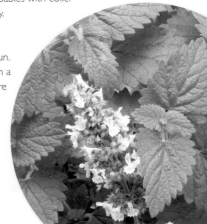

Lore and traditional uses

- In France, catnip is a traditional kitchen herb, as the leaves and young shoots are used to season, tenderize and marinade meats.
- Chewing the root is said to make even the most gentle person fierce and quarrelsome.

Enhancing mind and spirit

- To bring luck and happiness to your life, light powdered dried catnip leaves in an incense burner and waft the smoke around the room.

Caring for your body

- To melt away tension headaches, anxiety and insomnia, take 1 cup catnip infusion (see first preparation, right) up to three times daily.
- To soothe stress-related indigestion, take 1 tsp catnip tincture (see second preparation, right) up to three times daily, as required.
- To reduce fluid retention in the legs, apply a catnip leaf poultice (see p.23) to the affected areas, every morning and evening, until the swelling subsides.

Core benefits

Soothes anxiety

Mildly sedative

Regulates digestion

Preparations

Infusion: 1 tsp dried or 2 tsp fresh catnip flowering tops or leaves in 1 cup just-boiled water (put a lid on the cup during steeping). Standard method (p.20).

Tincture: 200g (7oz) dried or 400g (14oz) fresh catnip flowering tops or leaves in 1 litre (2 pints) vodka-water mix. Standard method (p.20).

Evening primrose *Oenothera biennis*

To watch the yellow flower of an evening primrose unfurl in the twilight is one of life's little treats; once it's dark you might even see the flower's mysterious emissions of phosphorescent light. The seed oil is the plant's true miracle-worker. It contains several fatty acids that the body needs for healthy skin, including gamma-linolenic acid (GLA), which also balances the female hormones, reduces allergic eczema and improves the circulation. New research shows that properties in evening primrose ease depression and hyperactivity, and reduce prostate swelling. The aerial parts are astringent, so soothing for coughs; and its roots may be used for bowel health.

Growing and harvesting

- Enjoys dryish, well-drained, sandy loam in sun.
- Sow seeds *in situ* in early summer.
- Harvest stem "skin", leaves and flowers in summer; dry. Harvest ripe seeds in autumn; dry, then grind or press out oil using a pestle and mortar. Dig up roots in second year; dry.

Plant type:
Hardy biennial

Description: 1m (3ft) high by 30cm (1ft) wide; tiny black seeds

Native habitat: Cool temperate; E North America

Parts of plant used: Seeds, roots, leaves, stem "skins", flowers

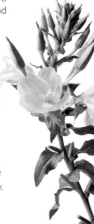

Lore and traditional uses
• Native North Americans used the plant's leaf poultice to heal bruises and hemorrhoids.

Enhancing mind and spirit
• To calm an erratic personality or relieve dementia, take 3–5g evening primrose oil, in capsules, three to five times daily, as needed.

Caring for your body
• To strengthen the heart against chronic stress and to lower blood pressure, take 1g evening primrose oil, in capsules, two to four times daily, as required.
• To soothe a spasmodic cough, take 1 cup evening primrose infusion (see first preparation, right) three times daily, until the cough has gone.
• To relieve premenstrual or menopausal symptoms, take 1g evening primrose oil, in capsules, three to five times daily.
• To assist a weight-loss plan, drink 1 cup evening primrose decoction (see second preparation, right) with every meal.

Core benefits
Relieves stress

Balances hormones

Improves circulation

Preparations

Infusion: 1 tsp dried evening primrose leaves and stem "skins" in 1 cup just-boiled water. Standard method (p.20).

Decoction 30g (1oz) dried evening primrose root in 750ml (1½ pints) water. Standard method (p.20).

211

Passionflower *Passiflora incarnata*

Spanish missionaries named this plant passionflower in the 16th century: the intricate markings on the flowers were thought to symbolize aspects of Christ's Passion. The leaves and stems provide a non-drowsy sedative for insomnia and anxiety, and can prevent a rapid heartbeat, reduce high blood pressure and relieve muscle tension. The leaves offer a remedy for nausea caused by drug withdrawal and reduce the brain's perception of nerve pain, easing the symptoms of neuralgia and shingles. Avoid passionflower during pregnancy.

Plant type: Half-hardy, ever-green perennial climber

Description: Up to 9m (30ft) tall; cream to laven-der flowers; edible fruits

Native habitat: All tropical; S América, southern USA

Parts of plant used: Leaves, stems, flowers, roots, fruit

Growing and harvesting

- Prefers well-drained, light, rich soil in full sun.
- In early spring, soak seeds for 12 hours in warm water, then surface-sow in a greenhouse. Or take 15cm (6in) cuttings in summer and plant in sandy soil.
- Harvest aerial parts in summer. Use fresh, or dry.

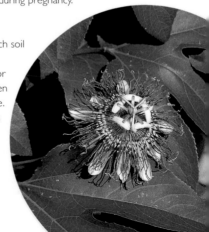

Lore and traditional uses

- Native Americans used the whole passionflower plant to treat swollen and irritated eyes, and the root as a general tonic.
- Mexicans traditionally take passionflower for insomnia, epilepsy and hysteria.

Enhancing mind and spirit

- To access higher levels of consciousness, put 4 drops passionflower flower essence (see pp.34–5) under the tongue before meditating.
- To treat stress-related insomnia, drink 1 cup passionflower "sweet sleep tea" (see first preparation, right) before bed, as required.

Caring for your body

- To lower stress-related high blood pressure, or ease heart palpitations or indigestion, take 1 cup passionflower leaf infusion (see second preparation, right) up to three times daily.
- To soothe minor skin irritations, make a compress (see p.23) using double-strength passionflower leaf infusion (see second preparation, right); apply to the affected areas.

Core benefits

Sedative

Lowers blood pressure

Soothes skin irritation

Preparations

Sweet sleep tea: Steep ½ tsp dried passion-flower leaf, ½ tsp dried blue skullcap leaf and ½ tsp dried valerian root in 1 cup just-boiled water for 10 minutes. Strain.

Infusion: ½–1 tsp dried passionflower leaves in 1 cup just-boiled water. Standard method (p.20). (For double strength, use 1–2 tsp dried leaves in 1 cup water.)

213

Cowslip *Primula veris*

The petals of this spring flower provide a soothing remedy for nervous tension and headaches, and an excellent sedative for over-excitement. They fight skin-aging free radicals, and so are also a tonic for acne and sunburn. The roots have an expectorant action on respiratory problems, such as chronic bronchitis, and contain an aspirin-like compound that eases pain. They also have anti-inflammatory properties to reduce the swelling and spasms of rheumatism and arthritis. Halve all dosages if you are pregnant or taking blood-thinning medication. The flowers' stamens may cause skin reactions on contact. Never pick this increasingly rare plant in the wild.

Growing and harvesting

- Prefers a light, well-drained, moist soil in sun.
- Sow seeds in summer when ripe. Or propagate by dividing mature plants some time between autumn and spring.
- Harvest flowers in late spring, then use fresh, or dry for later use. After first year, dig up roots in spring or autumn, then dry.

Plant type:
Hardy perennial

Description: 25cm (10in) high by 25cm (10in) wide; golden flowers; milky scent

Native habitat: Cool temperate; Europe, W Asia

Parts of plant used: Flowers, leaves, roots

Preparations

Infusion: 1 tsp dried or 2 tsp fresh cowslip flowers in 1 cup just-boiled water. Standard method (p.20). (For double strength, use 2 tsp dried or 4 tsp fresh flowers in 1 cup water.)

Tincture: 200g (7oz) dried cowslip root in 1 litre (2 pints) vodka-water mix. Standard method (p.20).

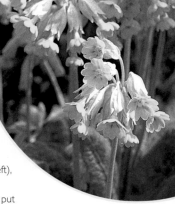

Lore and traditional uses

- According to 17th-century English herbalist Nicholas Culpeper, using a skin ointment containing cowslip will result in enhanced beauty.
- In Denmark, cowslip is a long-held remedy for convulsions.

Enhancing mind and spirit

- To soothe anxiety, take 1 cup cowslip flower infusion (see first preparation, left), as required.
- To restore a sense of playfulness in life, put 2 drops cowslip flower essence (see pp.34–5) in a glass of water and sip throughout the day.

Caring for your body

- To ease lung congestion, take 1 tsp cowslip tincture (see second preparation, left) three or four times daily.
- To rejuvenate the complexion, rinse the face with cooled, double-strength cowslip flower infusion (see first preparation, left) twice daily.

Core benefits

Soothes stress

Decongestant

Tones the skin

215

Blue skullcap *Scutellaria lateriflora*

In late summer the dry seed capsules of this pretty flower are a small cap shape, giving the herb its name. Blue skullcap's aerial parts are a restorative nerve tonic for all types of anxiety and stress, as they soothe both the muscles and the nervous system – often calming nerves within 30 minutes. They can also help reduce the symptoms of withdrawal from some drugs (including alcohol and barbiturates), improve bloodflow in the brain and reduce muscle spasm. Avoid taking blue skullcap during pregnancy.

Plant type:
Hardy perennial

Description: 1m (3ft) high by 60m (2ft) wide; tubular purple-blue flowers

Native habitat: Cool temperate; N America, Europe

Parts of plant used:
Flowers, leaves, stems, roots

Growing and harvesting

- Grows in a cool, moist site, in part shade.
- Sow seeds *in situ* in late spring.
- Harvest leaves or whole flowering tops in midsummer. The leaves are best used fresh or in a tincture as their potency decreases slightly with age.

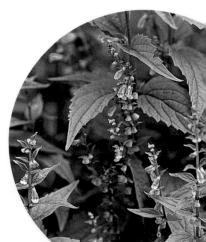

216

Lore and traditional uses

- Cherokee Native North Americans smoked blue skullcap ceremonially to induce visions, while the Iroquois used skullcap root infusion to keep the throat clear.

Enhancing mind and spirit

- To calm nervous anxiety, depression and insomnia, mix ½ cup blue skullcap infusion (see first preparation, right) with ½ cup lemon balm leaf infusion (see p.206) and drink up to three times a day, as needed.
- To induce visionary dreams, put 1 tsp powdered blue skullcap leaves on an incense disk while meditating before sleep.

Caring for your body

- To reduce symptoms of withdrawal (from any addiction), take 2 or 3 size 00 capsules filled with powdered blue skullcap leaf (see p.21) three times daily.
- To help relieve rheumatic or neuralgia pain, take 1 tsp blue skullcap tincture (see second preparation, right) three times daily.

Core benefits

Relaxes the nerves

Eases withdrawal

Relieves pain

Preparations

Infusion: 2 tsp fresh blue skullcap flowering tops in 1 cup just-boiled water. Standard method (p.20).

Tincture: 400g (14oz) fresh blue skullcap flowering tops in 1 litre (2 pints) vodka-water mix. Standard method (p.20).

217

Linden *Tilia* species

Linden – or lime – trees often have flowers so fragrant that a single tree can scent an entire street. Lime blossoms (as the flowers are most commonly known) are brewed to make a digestive infusion, as well as to treat insomnia and nervous stress, and over-anxiety in children. The infusion also induces sweating, helping to remove toxins from the body, and reduces headaches, the symptoms of colds and flu, and high blood pressure. You can apply the flower water externally as a skin tonic for rashes, freckles and wrinkles, and use it in the bath to soothe rheumatic aches, or even to calm fractious children.

Growing and harvesting
- Prefers a good moist, loamy soil and sun.
- Grow from very fresh seed (not more than a week old). Be patient – germination can take up to 18 months.
- Harvest blossoms in midsummer with their winged bract (leaf-like outer casing). Dry in a warm, dark place. Keep for up to 9 months: stale, old flowers may cause mild intoxication.

Plant type: Hardy deciduous tree

Description: 40m (130ft) tall by 25m (80ft) wide; tiny, fragrant cream flowers

Native habitat: Cool temperate; Europe

Parts of plant used: Leaves, stems, roots, seeds, timber, sapwood

Preparations

Infusion: 1 tsp dried or 2 tsp fresh lime blossoms in 1 cup just-boiled water. Standard method (p.20).

Tincture: 200g (7oz) dried or 400g (14oz) fresh lime blossoms in 1 litre (2 pints) vodka-water mix. Standard method (p.20).

Lore and traditional uses
- In Greek myth, the Titan Kronos disguised himself as a horse to rape the nymph Philyra. To free the nymph from her shame, the gods turned her into a linden tree.
- In France, emollient lime blossoms are used in skin lotions.

Enhancing mind and spirit
- To relax nervous excitability, take 1 cup lime blossom infusion (see first preparation, left) up to three times daily.
- To calm hyperactivity in children, add 2 litres (4 pints) lime blossom infusion (see first preparation, left) to their bedtime bath.

Caring for your body
- To expel catarrh or relieve congestion, take 1 tsp linden tincture (see second preparation, left) three or four times daily.
- To soothe itchy skin, apply lime blossom infused oil (see p.23) to the affected area.

Core benefits

Calms the nerves

Expels catarrh

Lowers blood pressure

Valerian *Valeriana officinalis*

Valerian is the most widely used sedative in Europe. Its unskinned root is excellent for nervous overstrain – with none of the side-effects of conventional medicine. The whole herb is used internally to treat muscle cramps and irritable bowel syndrome, and topically for wounds, ulcers and eczema. Don't take valerian for more than six weeks at a time before breaking for a week, then resuming if necessary.

Plant type:
Hardy perennial

Description: 1m (3ft) high by 60cm (2ft) wide; pale pink flowers

Native habitat: Cool temperate; Europe, W Asia

Parts of plant used: Leaves, roots, rhizome, essential oil (from rhizome)

Growing and harvesting
- Prefers moist, loamy soil in light shade.
- Sow seeds in spring in a seed tray. Or divide mature plants in spring.
- Harvest two-year-old rhizomes and roots once leaves have died. Use fresh, or dry.

Lore and traditional uses
- Valerian was used during World War I to treat shell-shock and again during World War II to soothe air-raid stress.

220

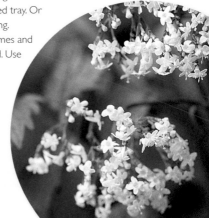

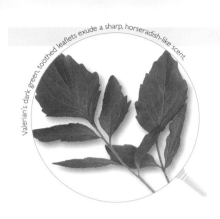

Valerian's dark green, toothed leaflets exude a sharp, horseradish-like scent.

Enhancing mind and spirit

- To calm overwrought nerves, take 1 cup valerian root infusion (see first preparation, right) up to three times daily.

Caring for your body

- To reduce high blood pressure, take ½–1 tsp valerian tonic wine (see second preparation, right) up to three times daily, as needed.
- To soothe anxiety-related pre-menstrual syndrome, take up to 3 size 00 capsules filled with powdered valerian root (see p.21) three times daily, as required.
- To draw out a splinter, apply a compress soaked in double-strength valerian infusion (see first preparation, right) twice daily.

Preparations

Infusion: Crush 1 tsp fresh valerian root and soak it for 12–24 hours in 1 cup cool water; strain, then drink. (For double strength, use 2 tsp fresh root in 1 cup cool water.)

Tonic wine: Wash 50g (1¾oz) fresh valerian root, then sun-dry for 2 hours. Crush and add to 1 cup acidic white wine. Steep for 1 month.

CHAPTER 8

Romantic Aphrodisiacs

This chapter brims with herbs that act on the mind, body and spirit to encourage intimacy and romance in your life, and to spark sensual desire.

Some of the herbs have been selected because of their historical or legendary associations as symbols of love. For example, sweet myrtle is associated with Aphrodite, the Greek goddess of love; orange blossom is a traditional bridal flower to represent purity; and the rose, of course, is the ultimate symbol of romance. The effects of these herbs on the body support their romantic associations by soothing the mind, encouraging trust, and reducing inhibitions.

When seeking to inspire romance, there is nothing more alluring than scent. Flowers such as jasmine, henna and the Madonna lily have rich, narcotic perfumes to suggest exotic mystery and adventure. The spices, including coriander and vanilla, are warm and

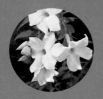 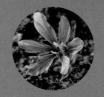 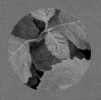

stimulating. They boost the circulation, enhancing arousal and inviting playful contact – these herbs are the key ingredients in sensuous foods and enticing love potions.

Earthy scents, from vetiver, patchouli and saffron, will encourage a deeper connection with your lover, enveloping you both in their reassuring, comforting qualities.

Sheer animal desire is roused by herbs that have a muskiness to their scents.

Blackcurrant has a directly erotic, almost feral, odour that can be unpleasant on its own, but blended in tiny amounts with other fragrances gives an undercurrent of arousal. Meanwhile, properties in damiana and ashwagandha will help restore libido and boost sexual potency.

Use your romantic herbs to make your own love potions, room sprays, perfumes or massage oils – and, above all, enjoy your experiments!

Bitter orange *Citrus aurantium*

The scent of the blossom of the bitter orange tree – sweet and clean, but also luxurious – has a long connection with romance and weddings, as the white flowers represent purity and chastity and their haunting fragrance can relax an apprehensive bride. Orange blossom essential oil (known as neroli after a 17th-century Italian princess from Nerola, who used the oil to scent her gloves) is a highly prized aphrodisiac oil, often used in perfumery. Applied topically, diluted in a carrier oil (see p.27), neroli helps rejuvenate mature skin cells.

Plant type:
Evergreen tree

Description: 6m (20ft) tall by 6m (20ft) wide; fragrant white flowers

Native habitat: Tropical grassland; S Europe, SE Asia

Parts of plant used: Leaves, flowers, stems, fruit, seeds, essential oil (from flowers, leaves and twigs)

Growing and harvesting

- Prefers well-drained, medium-loamy soil in full sun.
- Rinse ripe seed (taken after fruit ripens). Sow in spring, or in a greenhouse any time. Or take flexible cuttings in late summer.
- Harvest flowers when they open in late spring. Use fresh, or dry.

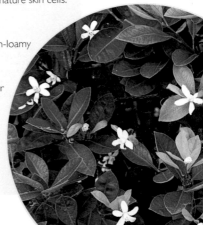

Lore and traditional uses

• In England in the 19th century, orange blossoms were woven into bridal bouquets as a symbol of the bride's purity.

• In aromatherapy, neroli is used traditionally to relieve anxiety, improve circulation and heal thread veins, scars and stretchmarks.

Enhancing mind and spirit

• To soothe away nervous apprehension before a romantic encounter, take 1 cup bitter orange blossom infusion (see first preparation, right).

Caring for your body

• To regenerate skin cells, rejuvenating the skin, or to reduce stretchmarks and thread veins, massage a few drops of neroli blend (see second preparation, right) into affected areas on the face or body twice daily.

• To speed up resting metabolic rate, take 1 tsp unripe peel tincture (available commercially) three times daily, and massage the body with 1 drop neroli in 1 tsp sweet almond oil.

Core benefits

Boosts confidence

Rejuvenates the skin

Optimizes metabolism

Preparations

Infusion: 1–2 tsp dried or 2–3 tsp fresh orange blossoms in 1 cup just-boiled water. Standard method (p.20).

Neroli blend: Blend 3 drops neroli, 4 drops rose and 3 drops frankincense essential oils in 4 tsp jojoba oil.

225

Coriander *Coriandrum sativum*

In the Middle Ages, the seed of this aromatic annual was a popular ingredient in love potions, among them the medicinal spiced wine *hipocras*, which aimed to increase the circulation and stimulate the libido, as well as to provide a digestive tonic. Coriander seed is mildly narcotic, and develops a sweet, spicy flavour as it ripens. This flavour is intensified by drying. Herbalists use coriander leaves (also known as cilantro) to relieve irritated skin and as a tonic for the brain and nervous system.

Plant type:
Annual

Description: 45cm (1½ft) high by 30cm (1ft) wide; tiny white flowers

Native habitat: Warm temperate; W Asia, N Africa

Parts of plant used: Seeds, leaves, stems, roots, essential oil (from seeds and leaves)

Growing and harvesting

- Sow in warm, dry soil in sun after last frost or, for more leaf production, sow in a little shade.
- Harvest leaves any time, and use fresh. Pick ripe seeds in late summer, then dry.

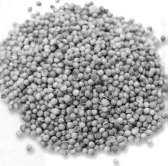

Lore and traditional uses

- In Traditional Chinese Medicine, coriander is used as a longevity herb, while in Indian Ayurvedic medicine

it is digestive and detoxifying and enhances natural defences against allergens.

- Roman legions carried coriander on their conquests through Europe, using the herb to flavour bread. The Romans also used coriander mixed with cumin and vinegar to preserve meat.

Enhancing mind and spirit

- To intensify affection between you and your partner, end a romantic meal with a small glass of *hipocras* (see first preparation, right).
- To encourage a romantic atmosphere in the bedroom, mist-spray your bed linen with a blend of 3 drops coriander essential oil in 2 tbsp rose water.

Caring for your body

- To sweeten your breath, rinse your mouth with ½ cup cooled coriander decoction (see second preparation, right).
- To speed up healing of skin and mouth ulcers, apply a paste of 1 tsp coriander seed powder mixed into a few drops of olive oil.

Core benefits

Stimulating

Sweetens breath

Aids digestion

Preparations

Hipocras: Bring to a boil 1 litre (2 pints) red wine and 1 cup honey. Off the heat, add 1 tsp each coriander seed, ginger, cinnamon, cardamom, white pepper, clove, nutmeg and caraway seed, and 1 cup rose petals. Stir, leave for 24 hours, strain. Mature for 6 weeks.

Decoction: Boil 1 tsp seed in 1½ cups water for 5–10 minutes. Strain.

227

Saffron *Crocus sativus*

Between the petals of the saffron crocus
– which stays open day and night – dangle
three thread-like, vermilion stigmas. These
become the sweet, earthy-flavoured saffron
spice featured in many aromatic dishes. Saffron's
cordial effect on the brain and heart give the
plant its romantic reputation. The Arabs once
mixed saffron with henna and rubbed it into
a bride's skin for its seductive scent. Herbalists
use saffron to ease fevers and cramps and
reduce enlarged livers, and to calm nerves. It
will speed up healing of bruises, and ease the
discomfort of rheumatic and neuralgia pain.

Plant type: Hardy corm
(bulb-like)

Description: 15cm (6in)
high by 8cm (3in) wide;
single mauve flower

Native habitat: Warm temperate; Greece, Asia Minor

Parts of plant used:
Flower stigmas

Growing and harvesting

- Grows in well-drained, loamy soil
  in sun.
- Propagate by corm division.
  Plant 12cm (5in) deep in
  summer.
- Pick stigmas when flowers
  open mid-autumn. Dry
  for 2–3 days in absorbent
  paper in a cupboard.

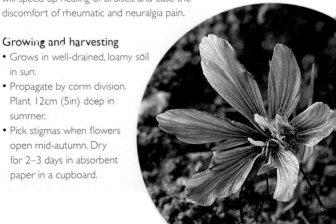

Lore and traditional uses

- According to Greek lore, a girl who ate saffron for a week would not be able to resist a potential lover.
- In Indian Ayurvedic medicine, saffron improves sexual potency, menstruation, blood circulation and energy levels.

Enhancing mind and spirit

- To boost energy in the morning or revive you after a tiring day, drink a cup of *qahwa* tea (see first preparation, right).
- To overcome nervous tension, insomnia or depression, take ½ cup saffron milk infusion (see second preparation, right) up to three times daily, for as long as necessary.

Caring for your body

- To enhance sexual potency in men, take 1 cup of saffron water infusion (see second preparation, right), a mouthful at a time, every day.
- To improve digestion, drink 1 cup *qahwa* tea (see first preparation, right) after a meal.

Core benefits

Improves libido

Strengthens the nerves

Aids digestion

Preparations

Qahwa (Kashmiri tea): Brew ½ tsp green tea in 2 cups water; add 3 saffron threads, 1 crushed cardamom seed, ⅛ tsp ground cinnamon and 2½ tsp shredded almonds. Reheat, sweeten and drink.

Infusion: Steep 12 saffron threads in 1 cup just-boiled milk or water for 7 minutes. Strain, then drink.

229

Jasmine *Jasminum officinale*

Known as "Queen of the Night", jasmine is planted around courtyards, verandas and windows for its intoxicating evening perfume. The flowers have an engaging fresh, green undertone and provide a potent aphrodisiac. They can help boost sexual confidence in both sexes and increase sperm production in men, as well as spiritualizing and enhancing intimacy in a sexual relationship. Jasmine essential oil has a potent fragrance, so it is best used only in tiny amounts.

Plant type: Evergreen vine, but can be trained to shrub

Description: Up to 10m (30ft) long; highly fragrant white flowers

Native habitat: All tropical; Asia

Parts of plant used: Flowers, leaves, roots, essential oil (from flowers)

Growing and harvesting

- Enjoys a well-drained loamy soil with high levels of light and humidity; tolerates shade on a warm site.
- Sow seeds when ripe in a greenhouse. Grow in small pots; protect from frost. Alternatively, take flexible cuttings in summer.
- Pick summer flowers before dawn. Use fresh (for the best scent), or dry.

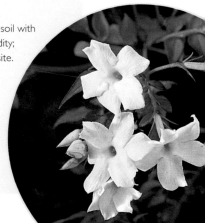

Lore and traditional uses

- In Ayurvedic medicine, jasmine flowers are prescribed to reduce fevers and fortify the immune system.
- Throughout Asia, jasmine flowers are given as temple offerings and used to scent hair.

Enhancing mind and spirit

- To evoke soothing reassurance for deep, unsettling emotions, or to create an atmosphere of intimacy with your partner, give and receive a massage using a few drops of jasmine flower infused oil (see p.23).

Caring for your body

- To rejuvenate the skin, apply jasmine skin gel (see first preparation, right) daily.
- To relieve aching muscles or rheumatic pain, hold a compress (see p.23) made with single-strength jasmine flower infusion (see second preparation, right) against the affected area.
- To scent long hair with aromatic jasmine, wrap the hair around fresh jasmine flowers and leave it in place for three hours.

Core benefits

Promotes desire

Alleviates stress

Painkilling

Preparations

Skin gel: Stir 2 drops jasmine essential oil into 2 tbsp aloe vera gel. Scoop into small, clean jar, seal, and refrigerate for up to 1 month.

Single-strength infusion: 1 tsp dried or 2 tsp fresh jasmine flowers in 1 cup just-boiled water. Standard method (p.20).

231

Henna *Lawsonia inermis*

As Cleopatra approached the waiting Mark Antony, a breeze of fragrance announced her arrival: she had had the sails of her barge soaked in *cyprinum*, her seductive henna flower perfume. Henna flowers are still available today on the streets of Cairo. The leaves yield the famous red dye used to stain bodies, hair and drums, but herbalists use them for their cooling astringency, which soothes fevers, headaches and skin irritations.

Plant type:
Evergreen shrub

Description: 6m (20ft) high by 6m (20ft) wide; fragrant small cream flowers

Native habitat: Tropical grassland; N Africa, S Asia

Parts of plant used: Flowers, leaves, roots, fruit, bark, seeds, essential oil (from flowers)

Growing and harvesting
- Grow in well-drained soil in sun.
- Sow ripe seeds in autumn outdoors in Tropics, otherwise indoors in spring.
- Pick flowers in early summer and use fresh; pick leaves just before flowering, then use fresh, or dry.

Lore and traditional uses
- Nubians (from southern Egypt) carried deodorizing henna leaves in their

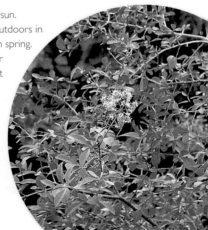

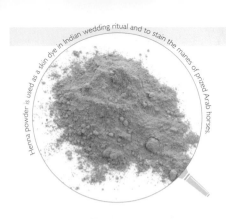

Henna powder is used as a skin dye in Indian wedding ritual and to stain the manes of prized Arab horses.

Core benefits

Alluring

Nerve tonic

Soothing

armpits to mask body odour. The Romans used the leaves to treat smelly feet.

Enhancing mind and spirit

- To fragrance a room for a romantic encounter, mist-spray the air with 4 drops henna essential oil in 4 tsp water.
- To promote deep sleep, take 1 tsp henna tincture (see first preparation, right).

Caring for your body

- To reduce muscular aches, massage with henna flower infused oil (see p.23) twice daily.
- To soothe a fever, take 1 cup henna leaf infusion (see second preparation, right) up to three times daily.

Preparations

Tincture: 200g (7oz) dried or 400g (14oz) fresh henna leaves in 1 litre (2 pints) vodka-water mix. Standard method (p.20).

Infusion: 1 tsp dried or 2 tsp fresh henna leaves in 1 cup just-boiled water. Standard method (p.20).

233

Madonna lily *Lilium candidum*

The Madonna lily has many spiritual connections. In Christianity, for example, it represents purity, chastity and innocence, while in Eastern religions it denotes fertility. In medieval Europe, the flower was a main ingredient in magical potions prescribed to attract a lover. The flower's emollient qualities (captured in an oil infusion) help improve the skin's texture and heal eczema. The bulbs were once boiled and eaten as a food, but they also contain a soothing mucilage, valued in creams to treat burns, boils and acne.

Growing and harvesting

- Prefers well-drained, fertile soil in sun.
- Best grown from bulbs. In late summer, plant 2.5cm (1in) below soil level.
- Flowers in summer: pick whole flowers and use fresh, or freeze. Dig up bulb in late summer; use fresh, or dry.

Plant type:
Hardy bulb

Description: 1.5m (5m) high by 45cm (1½ft) wide; fragrant white flowers

Native habitat: Warm temperate; Balkans, W Asia

Parts of plant used:
Flowers, bulb, essential oil (from flowers)

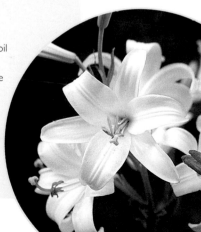

234

Lore and traditional uses

- In Greek myth, the lily was created when milk from the goddess Hera's breast spilled on the floor as she nursed the infant hero Herakles.
- Persian women bathed with Madonna lily essential oil to maintain their youthful beauty.

Enhancing mind and spirit

- To release self-judgment and liberate inhibitions within a relationship, put 2 drops Madonna lily flower essence (see pp.34–5) in 1 cup water and sip throughout the day.

Caring for your body

- To moisturize skin, reduce wrinkles and improve skin texture, apply Madonna lily skin cream (see first preparation, right) twice daily.
- To reduce thread veins and heal bruises, dab the affected areas with Madonna lily tincture (see second preparation, right) twice daily.
- To reduce tumours, skin ulcers, boils and acne, mash a Madonna lily bulb and use it to make a poultice (see p.23). Apply to the affected areas two or three times daily, as required.

Core benefits

Promotes intimacy

Rejuvenates the skin

Reduces inflammation

Preparations

Skin cream: Juice 1 Madonna lily bulb and add to 1 tbsp honey and 30g (1oz) beeswax in a bowl over a pan of boiling water. Stir until melted. Mix in 3–4 tbsp rose infusion (see p.243). Cool and store in jars.

Tincture: 400g (14oz) fresh Madonna lily flowers in 1 litre (2 pints) vodka-water mix. Standard method (p.20).

Sweet myrtle *Myrtus communis*

Associated with Aphrodite, the Greek goddess of love, sweet myrtle's ivory flowers are a traditional symbol of beauty, chastity and sensuality, often woven into bridal wreaths. The plant has a fresh, spicy-sweet orange-blossom scent. Its buds can be infused in alcohol to make "angel flower water", which, along with the plant's antiseptic leaves, is used in creams to help heal acne. The scent of the plant's leaves and branchlets makes them suitable for using in pot pourri and strewing as an insect repellent.

Growing and harvesting
- Succeeds in well-drained soil and sun.
- Soak seeds for 24 hours in warm water, then sow in late winter in a greenhouse. Or take 8cm (3in) flexible cuttings in midsummer. Protect from heavy frosts.
- Pick leaves anytime, then dry. Pick buds or flowers midsummer, then use fresh, or dry.

Lore and traditional uses
- Ayurvedic practitioners use sweet myrtle to treat cerebral problems, including epilepsy.

Plant type: Half-hardy evergreen shrub

Description: 5m (17ft) high by 3m (10ft) wide; creamy white flowers

Native habitat: Warm temperate; S Europe, N Africa

Parts of plant used: Flowers, leaves, fruit, essential oil (from leaves, twigs and flowers)

Preparations

Tincture: 200g (7oz) dried or 400g (14oz) fresh sweet myrtle flowers in 1 litre (2 pints) vodka-water mix. Standard method (p.20).

Decoction: 30g (1oz) dried or 60g (2oz) fresh sweet myrtle flowers in 750ml (1½ pints) water. Standard method (p.20).

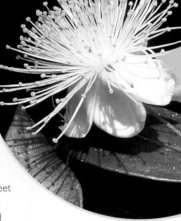

• In France, women traditionally drank sweet myrtle tea to slow down the aging process.

Enhancing mind and spirit
• To encourage self-worth and positive relationships, massage the body with sweet myrtle leaf infused oil (see p.23).

Caring for your body
• To refresh the skin, splash on 1 tsp sweet myrtle tincture diluted in 2 tbsp sweet myrtle decoction (see first and second preparations, left) twice daily.
• To relieve respiratory congestion, take 1 cup sweet myrtle decoction (see second preparation, left) up to three times daily.

Special tip
To impart a sweet-smoky flavour to barbecue meats, dip a few sweet myrtle leaves and branchlets in water and lay them under the meats for the final 10 minutes' cooking time.

Core benefits

Relaxes the emotions

Cleanses the skin

Relieves congestion

237

Patchouli *Pogostemon cablin*

The earthy, musky aroma from the leaves of this nettle-like plant has given patchouli its status as an aphrodisiac, and it is often used in southeast Asian love potions. The same scent may be used in herbalism to relieve stress and repel insects. The plant's leaves and stems have antiseptic, stimulant and antidepressant properties, and in southeast Asia they are used to counter snake bites. Patchouli's essential oil regenerates skin cells, helping to heal cracked skin, and makes an aromatic treatment for oily hair and dandruff.

Plant type:
Perennial

Description: 1m (3ft) high by 1m (3ft) wide; small white flowers

Native habitat: Tropical rainforest; SE Asia, India

Parts of plant used:
Leaves, stems, essential oil (from leaves)

Growing and harvesting

- Requires rich, moist but well-drained soil in sun or partial shade.
- If available, sow the tiny, fragile seeds in spring. Alternatively, take cuttings in late spring, or divide the rootball (mass of roots) in autumn.
- Harvest leaves throughout summer. Use fresh, or dry.

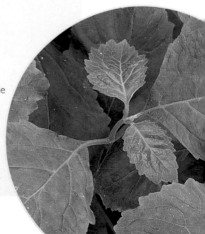

Lore and traditional uses

- In the 18th and 19th centuries, silk traders from China put patchouli leaves inside their silks to deter moths. The scent became an indicator of true "Oriental" fabric – so much so that French and English cloth had to be similarly scented to secure buyers.

Enhancing mind and spirit

- To cement a positive, sensual connection with your lover, give each other a back and shoulder massage using a few drops patchouli massage blend (see first preparation, right).
- To ease nervous exhaustion, pour 1 litre (2 pints) patchouli leaf infusion (see second preparation, right) into a warm bath and relax in it for 20 minutes.

Caring for your body

- To reduce wrinkles, blend 2 drops jasmine essential oil in 3 tsp patchouli leaf infused oil (see p.23) and apply to the face twice daily.
- To relieve the itching of insect bites or stings, chew a patchouli leaf and apply it as required.

Core benefits

Stimulates desire

Relaxes the nerves

Supports the skin

Preparations

Massage blend: Mix 2 drops patchouli and 5 drops sweet orange essential oils in 4 tsp rose-petal infused oil (see p.23 for how to make an infused oil).

Infusion: 1 tsp dried or 2 tsp fresh patchouli leaves in 1 cup just-boiled water. Standard method (p.20).

Blackcurrant *Ribes nigrum*

A musky scent gives a perfume its erogenous edge. This scent was once derived from animal glands, but now we have plant sources, one of which is blackcurrant. This plant's green, foxy note is extracted from its flower buds. In addition, the berries contain more vitamin C than oranges; the pressed seed oil has the same hormone-regulating benefits as borage (see p.198) and the leaves contain compounds that help the body detoxify. French chemists have found that blackcurrant leaf infusion draws toxins out of the body's tissues and stimulates the liver to expel them.

Plant type: Hardy deciduous shrub

Description: 2m (6ft) high by 2m (6ft) wide; greenish white flowers

Native habitat: Cool temperate; N Europe, Himalaya

Parts of plant used: Leaves, buds, roots, berries, seeds essential oil (from buds)

Growing and harvesting

- Grows in well-drained, but moist, loamy soil in sun.
- Sow ripe seeds in autumn in a greenhouse. Or take 15cm (6in) flexible cuttings in summer.
- Pick leaves in spring, then use fresh, or dry. Harvest fruit when ripe in late summer and use fresh; harvest buds in spring.

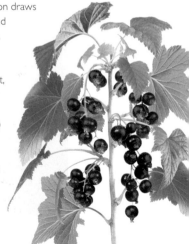

Lore and traditional uses
- The 18th-century French doctor Abbé Bailly believed blackcurrant's muskiness to be so potent that when he prescribed the herb he added a warning about its aphrodisiac effects.

Enhancing mind and spirit
- To keep the mind young or boost emotional sensitivity, take 1 cup blackcurrant leaf infusion (see first preparation, right) every morning.

Caring for your body
- To detoxify the skin cells and enhance the functions of the liver, kidneys and urinary tract, take 1 cup blackcurrant leaf infusion (see first preparation, right) three or four times daily, whenever you feel the need for a cleanse.
- To soothe away a child's cold or flu symptoms or sore throat, give 1 tsp blackcurrant cordial (see second preparation, right) in 1 cup water three times daily until the infection has gone.
- To repel insects or to soothe an insect bite, take a handful of blackcurrant leaves and rub them over your skin.

Core benefits
Heightens sensitivity

Detoxifies the cells

Relieves colds

Preparations

Infusion: Infuse 1 tbsp dried or 2 tbsp fresh blackcurrant leaves in 1 cup just-boiled water for 10 minutes. Strain, then drink.

Cordial: Juice ½ cup blackcurrants and mix with ½ cup stevia syrup (see p.124). Refrigerate for up to 1 week. (Adjust the amount of stevia syrup to taste, if necessary.)

241

Rose *Rosa officinalis*

A universal symbol of love, with a fragrance
that elicits a heart-opening smile, rose is a
romantic stimulant that uplifts and enfolds.
There are hundreds of species of rose, but *Rosa
officinalis* is sometimes called the "Apothecary's
rose", as it was the species grown in medieval
monastery gardens for medicinal purposes.
All parts of the rose plant are useful: rose
hips provide immunity-boosting vitamin C; the
leaves, a laxative; and beautiful rose essential oil,
a rejuvenating skin tonic and mood-enhancer.
The by-product of creating rose essential oil
is rose water, which is able to revive tired skin.

Plant type:
Deciduous shrub

Description: 1.5m (5ft)
high by 1.5m (5ft) wide;
deep pink flowers

Native habitat: All
temperate; S and C Europe

Parts of plant used:
Flowers, leaves, hips,
essential oil (from petals)

Growing and harvesting

• Prefers deep, well-drained soil,
  in sun after first year.
• Propagate from 25cm (8in)
  flexible cuttings in summer.
  Grow in wind-free shade
  for 12 months.
• Harvest flowers at their
  peak in summer, then use
  petals fresh, or dry.

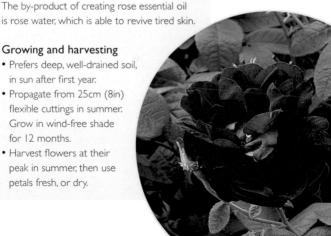

Lore and traditional uses

- The ancient Romans floated rose petals in their wine and beers as an aphrodisiac, and sprinkled rose petals on the marriage bed.

Enhancing mind and spirit

- To recapture deep tenderness with a lover, scent both partners' pillowcases with rose petals (see first preparation, right).
- To soothe grief, depression or insomnia, add 2 drops rose essential oil to a warm bath and rest in it for 20 minutes.

Caring for your body

- To rejuvenate mature skin and reduce thread veins, stir 2 drops rose essential oil into a small pot of unscented face cream and apply twice daily, morning and night.
- To refresh tired skin and eyes, apply rose water to the face twice daily.
- To relieve a cold, fever or sore throat, take 1 cup rose petal infusion (see second preparation, right) three times daily until the infection has gone.

Core benefits

Inspires romance

Tones the skin

Relieves infection

Preparations

Rose-scented pillow: Lay an empty pillowcase flat and cover one half with fragrant rose petals. Loosely fold over the other half and leave for 2–3 days in darkness. Discard the petals before inserting the pillows.

Infusion: Steep 1 tsp dried or 2 tsp fresh rose petals in 1 cup just-boiled water for 5 minutes. Strain; drink.

Damiana *Turnera aphrodisiaca*

In the 17th century, a Spanish missionary reported that Native Americans in Mexico drank damiana leaf tea to enhance lovemaking, a use dating back to the ancient Maya. Damiana leaves are credited with a wide range of tonic and stress-reducing virtues, with no toxic side-effects. They help restore libido by lowering anxiety and boosting circulation and energy, and may also treat mild depression, improve digestion and reduce constipation. The *Turnera diffusa* species of damiana has similar healing properties to those of *T. aphrodisiaca*.

Plant type: Small deciduous shrub

Description: 2m (7ft) high by 1.5m (5ft) wide; small, yellow summer flowers

Native habitat: Tropical rainforest; C and S America

Parts of plant used: Leaves, flowering tops

Growing and harvesting

- Needs dry soil and a sheltered position in sun.
- Sow seeds in spring, or take flexible cuttings in summer. Grow in a greenhouse for a year, then move outside; protect from frost.
- Pick leaves in summer during flowering. Use fresh, or dry in cool shade.

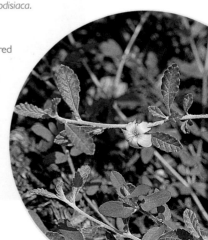

Lore and traditional uses

- Damiana appeared in the USA's *National Formulary* (a manual of approved medicine) as an aphrodisiac and a laxative.
- Germans have long taken damiana leaves as a tonic for the hormone and nervous systems.

Enhancing mind and spirit

- To cope with stress, depression and anxiety, take 1 cup damiana leaf infusion (see first preparation, right) two or three times daily.

Caring for your body

- To boost romantic energy and enhance sexual potency in both men and women, take 1 cup damiana leaf infusion (see first preparation, right), as required.
- To soothe a nervous digestive system, take 2 or 3 size 00 capsules filled with powdered damiana leaf (see p.21) up to three times daily, as required.
- To stimulate all the body's systems, take 1 tsp damiana tincture (see second preparation, right) three times daily, as required.

Core benefits

Boosts libido

Nerve tonic

Aids digestion

Preparations

Infusion: 1 tsp dried or 2 tsp fresh damiana leaves in 1 cup just-boiled water. Standard method (p.20).

Tincture: 200g (7oz) dried or 400g (14oz) fresh damiana leaves in 1 litre (2 pints) vodka-water mix. Standard method (p.20).

Vanilla *Vanilla planifolia*

According to research, whether it is worn as a perfume or eaten, vanilla ranks first of all nature's aphrodisiacs. It is not the fragrant flowers of this tropical orchid that commit the seduction, but the unripe beans, which are "cured" to develop their creamy, inviting aroma. Vanilla is also a digestive and, by boosting levels of adrenaline (epinephrine), an energizer.

Plant type:
Tropical vine

Description: Up to 15m (50ft) long; waxy white fragrant flowers

Native habitat: Tropical rainforest; C and S America

Parts of plant used:
Green bean pods

Growing and harvesting
• Requires rich soil in hot, humid shade.
• Take 1.5m (5ft) cuttings any time; leave to lie loosely coiled in dry shade for two weeks. Place base end in compost and train the rest as a loop to produce shoots and roots where the loop touches the ground.
• Pick beans when ripe (6 months). Then scald, ferment, and dry to cure.

Lore and traditional uses
• The Totonaca of Mexico, who first cultivated the

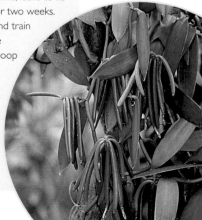

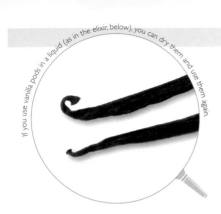

If you use vanilla pods in a liquid (as in the elixir, below), you can dry them and use them again.

Enhances intimacy

Restores the nerves

Stimulating

vanilla plant, rubbed vanilla bean oil on their skin until their bodies glistened.

Enhancing mind and spirit

- To exhilarate the brain and stimulate sexual energy, take 1 sherry glassful vanilla elixir (see first preparation, right), as required.
- To welcome your guests into a relaxing, comforting atmosphere, spray the room with vanilla room spray (see second preparation, right) just before they are due to arrive.

Caring for your body

- To stimulate your gastric juices, put ½ tsp vanilla essence in a small glass of pure water and drink before your evening meal.

Preparations

Vanilla elixir: Put 4 vanilla pods and a handful of rose petals in a glass jar and pour over 2 cups brandy. Soak for 4 weeks, shaking daily, then strain.

Room spray: In an atomizer, blend ½ tsp vanilla essence with 4 tsp water.

247

Vetiver *Vetiveria zizanioides*

Vetiver is a tall grass that grows in clumps. It has aromatic roots that tangle underground, helping to hold together the shifting soils on the hillsides where it is grown. The herb's reputation as an aphrodisiac comes from its green, woody scent, which enhances the sensuality of the body and reduces mental tension. Compounds in the root are said to stimulate the body's production of red blood cells, increasing oxygen in all the body's systems. They also lessen rheumatic pain and repel insects. The essential oil is a well-known relaxant.

Plant type:
Perennial grass

Description: 2m (7ft) tall; aromatic roots that can grow to 4m (13ft) deep

Native habitat: Tropical rainforest; Asia

Parts of plant used: Roots, essential oil (from roots)

Growing and harvesting
- Grow on deep, sandy loam in sun.
- Sow seeds in spring; or propagate by dividing mature plants in autumn. Always protect vetiver from frost.
- Harvest roots once they are two years old. Wash, clean and dry.

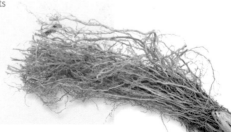

Lore and traditional uses

- In African-American folk magic, vetiver is said to attract good fortune, such as love and wealth, and repel bad luck.
- In India, vetiver roots are used to weave traditional fans, blinds and mats.

Enhancing mind and spirit

- To root the self in sensuality and reduce relationship anxiety, massage your body with a vetiver essential oil sensual blend (see first preparation, right).

Caring for your body

- To deeply nourish mature skin, reduce wrinkles and improve skin elasticity, apply vetiver skin gel (see second preparation, right) to the face and neck each morning.

Special tip

To scent your clothes and repel clothes moths, sew together two small squares of cotton, leaving an opening. Fill with chopped vetiver root, sew up, and place among stored clothes.

Core benefits

Increases sensuality

Reduces nervousness

Nourishes the skin

Preparations

Sensual blend: Blend 2 drops vetiver essential oil in 2 tsp sweet myrtle leaf infused oil (see p.237).

Skin gel: Blend 2 drops each vetiver, lavender and frankincense essential oils with 3 tbsp aloe gel (see p.173). Refrigerate in a clean jar for up to 1 month.

Ashwagandha *Withania somnifera*

Featured in the Indian epic the *Kama Sutra* (c.5th century CE) as a herb for heightening sexual experience, ashwagandha (or Indian ginseng) is used to restore male libido, cure impotence and increase sperm count. It may also increase female fertility. As an overall tonic, the root boosts vitality and helps the body better adapt to environmental and internal stress. Its antioxidant properties slow the aging process and enhance memory and clear thinking. The root is also a potent immunity-booster, often used to treat auto-immune problems, such as rheumatism. Never eat the aerial parts of the plant as they are toxic; and avoid taking the root during pregnancy.

Growing and harvesting

- Grow in well-drained, dryish soil in a warm, sheltered position in sun or dappled shade.
- Sow seeds in spring in a greenhouse (should germinate well in two weeks). Grow on in pots; move outside only after the last frost.
- Dig up three-year-old roots in autumn. Use fresh, or dry.

Plant type: Half-hardy, evergreen shrub

Description: 1m (3ft) high by 45cm (1½ft) wide; greenish or yellow flowers

Native habitat: Warm temperate; India, SE Asia

Parts of plant used: Roots, leaves, seeds

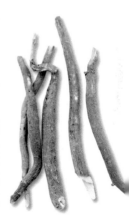

Lore and traditional uses

- In Indian Ayurvedic medicine, ashwagandha is a key restorative for stress and long-term illness and a sleep-inducer. It is also used to treat mental deficiency in the elderly.
- In Sri Lanka, ashwagandha leaves are used to repel insects.

Enhancing mind and spirit

- To enhance sexual vitality or restore libido, drink 1 cup ashwagandha decoction (see first preparation, right) up to three times daily for up to six weeks.
- To help the body adapt to stress and anxiety, and to improve memory and brain function, take ½ tsp ashwagandha tincture (see second preparation, right) three times daily, as required.

Caring for your body

- To reduce the inflammation of arthritis and rheumatism, take 2 or 3 size 00 capsules filled with powdered ashwagandha root (see p.21) three times daily, until symptoms improve.

Core benefits

Intensifies lovemaking

Alleviates stress

Improves brain function

Preparations

Decoction: 30g (1oz) dried ashwagandha root in 750ml (1½ pints) water. Standard method (p.20).

Tincture: 200g (7oz) dried ashwagandha root in 1 litre (2 pints) vodka-water mix. Standard method (p.20).

CHAPTER 9

Lifting the Spirit

This chapter is filled with herbs with rich, woody aromas that lift the spirits and encourage us along our spiritual path. Most of these plants are resinous trees, although there are a few other types, such as sagebrush, spikenard and clary sage, that share this spirit-lifting quality.

From earliest times, in all major cultures, people burned fragrant woods, roots and leaves to honour the gods and carry their prayers upward. Even today, the aromatic smoke of these plants will encourage you to breathe deeply, calming your mind, and, during meditation, helping your spirit to expand.

Traditionally, many resins were used as temple offerings, holy anointing oils, incense and perfume, as well as to scent clothes, bedding and private spaces. In this vein, the preparations in this chapter focus on making room

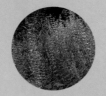
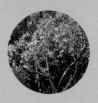

sprays, using vaporizers, and creating incense with powdered resin or leaves.

Incense is a wonderful way to enhance meditation, and many of the practical suggestions in this chapter encourage you to dip into meditation practice. Those who meditate may value the sense of peace it brings, but it also boosts levels of body chemicals associated with euphoria and self-confidence, and it fine-tunes the immune system, confirming the link between mind and body.

To burn incense safely, try to find charcoal incense disks made from specialist charcoal (not barbecue charcoal, which gives off noxious fumes). It's also a good idea to buy a traditional incense burner with three legs, as this will prevent the heat from damaging surfaces. The three legs represent mind, body and spirit – highlighting how aromatic incense uplifts on every level.

Aloe wood *Aquilaria agallocha*

I first came across mystical aloe wood in a temple in Kyoto. To inhale its unique, exotic, balsam aroma is to understand why it has been valued for 3,000 years as a perfume, an aphrodisiac and, most highly, a spiritual incense to awaken higher levels of consciousness. The fragrance is found only in trees with diseased heartwood, where resin collects to saturate the wood fibres. In Ayurvedic medicine, aloe wood is prescribed to reduce fever and inflammation, and support the nervous and respiratory systems, and as an aid to digestion.

Plant type:
Evergreen tree

Description: 40m (130ft) tall by 25m (80ft) wide; scented white flowers

Native habitat: Tropical rainforest; Asia

Part of plant used:
Diseased wood, essential oil (from wood)

Growing and harvesting

- Sow ripe seed in a heated greenhouse; keep well watered and shaded (the tree requires tropical conditions).
- Only one to seven percent of trees develop the disease or mutation that creates the aloe wood. It is possible to artificially induce the disease, but so far this gives inferior wood. The scent takes eight to 20 years to develop.

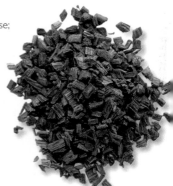

Lore and traditional uses

- For Buddhists, aloe wood transmutes ignorance into wisdom and calms the mind, while for Muslims it enhances Friday prayers.
- The Portuguese carved the wood into rosary beads, so the warmth of the hand would release the uplifting fragrance during prayers.

Enhancing mind and spirit

- To increase transcendent awareness during meditation, massage aloe wood hot-infused oil (see first preparation, right) into your upper body before you start.
- To bring clarity amid obsessive thinking or nervous exhaustion, wash your face and hair with aloe wood decoction (see second preparation, right), as required.

Caring for your body

- To ease indigestion, put 4–6 drops aloe wood essential oil in a bowl of just-boiled water. Lay a flannel over the surface of the water, then gently squeeze it out and rest with it on your abdomen for 20 minutes or more.

Core benefits

Nourishes spirituality

Revitalizes the mind

Aids digestion

Preparations

Hot-infused oil: Put 1 tbsp aloe wood chips and 1 cup grapeseed oil in a bowl over a pan of simmering water. Cover and leave for 2–3 hours. Cool and strain. Store for up to 9 months.

Decoction: 1 tbsp aloe wood chips or 2 tsp aloe wood powder in 750ml (1½ pints) water. Standard method (p.20).

Sagebrush *Artemisia tridentata*

In ceremonies, Native Americans smoulder the soft, silver aromatic leaves of this desert shrub for spiritual purification and protection. The smoke is remarkably calming. Sagebrush leaves improve digestion and are antiseptic. Used topically, they can prevent infection in wounds and sores and relieve pain.

Growing and harvesting
- Grow in dry, well-drained, lime-free soil in sun.
- Surface-sow seed in spring in a greenhouse; grow on in greenhouse over first winter. Or divide mature plants in spring or autumn.
- Pick sprigs from mature plants when in flower. Use fresh, or dry.

Lore and traditional uses
- Native American healers learn to recognize illness by connecting with the spirit of the sagebrush plant.
- Navajo Indians use sagebrush leaves to make a mouthwash and a

Plant type: Hardy evergreen shrub

Description: 3m (10ft) by 2m (7ft) wide; woolly white stems, silver leaves

Native habitat: Arid; Mexico, W USA

Parts of plant used: Flowering tops, leaves, essential oil (from flowering tops)

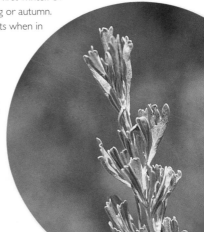

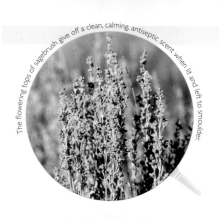

The flowering tops of sagebrush give off a clean, calming, antiseptic scent when lit and left to smoulder.

yellow fabric dye, as well as to protect food from insects and rodents.

Enhancing mind and spirit

- To cleanse your aura, light the tip of a smudge stick (see first preparation, right), then blow out the flame so the stick smoulders. Use your hand to draw smoke all around you.

Caring for your body

- To relieve a sore throat, gargle with 1 cup cooled sagebrush leaf infusion (see second preparation, right) up to three times daily.
- To aid the digestive system, take 1 cup sagebrush leaf infusion (see second preparation, right) three times daily.

Preparations

Smudge stick: Half-dry 3 juniper and 21 sagebrush sprigs. Strip leaves at base of stems and surround juniper with sagebrush. Tie together by winding string up then down. Secure at base. Dry for 3–7 days.

Infusion: 1 tsp dried or 2 tsp fresh sagebrush leaves in 1 cup just-boiled water. Standard method (p.20).

Frankincense *Boswellia sacra*

As early humans burned the gnarled stems
of this desert shrub, they would have noticed
the aromatic smoke, and the way it caused
their breathing to relax and their thoughts to
drift skyward. Frankincense was part of *kyphi*, a
blend of herbs and spices used in biblical Egypt
to enhance ritual and clear the emotions. The
resin is still valued today for spiritual exaltation,
and new research has found that its smoke
activates pathways in the brain to alleviate
anxiety. Furthermore, US research has found it
to be especially active against cancer cells and
the essential oil is a known skin rejuvenator.

Plant type:
Small evergreen tree

Description: 5m (16ft) tall
by 3m (10ft) wide; small
white flowers

Native habitat: Tropical dry;
Arabia, Yemen, Somalia

Parts of plant used:
Gum resin, essential oil
(from resin)

Growing and harvesting

- Grow in well-drained, dryish soil
  in full sun.
- Soak ripe seeds for five days
  in tepid water, then sow in a
  warm, dry greenhouse.
- Collect resin at the hottest
  times of year by making
  cuts in the bark of
  mature trees.

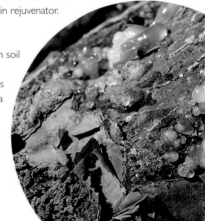

Lore and traditional uses

- The Egyptians charred frankincense resin and ground it into *kohl*, which they used as eyeliner and to maintain eye health.
- The 10th-century Persian physician Avicenna used frankincense to cure vomiting, diarrhea, fever and tumours.

Enhancing mind and spirit

- For deepened spiritual understanding, burn frankincense resin as an incense while meditating (see p.253).
- To melt away anxiety, blend 5 drops frankincense essential oil in 3 tsp sweet almond oil and massage into the body.

Caring for your body

- To restore dry or mature skin, or to reduce scarring (including acne scars), apply a few drops frankincense face oil (see first preparation, right) every evening before bed.
- To relieve lower back pain, rub frankincense hot-infused oil (see second preparation, right) into the affected area, as required.

Core benefits

Harmonizes the spirit

Rejuvenates the skin

Reduces inflammation

Preparations

Face oil: Blend 5 drops frankincense, 3 drops lavender and 2 drops sandalwood essential oils in 4 tsp jojoba oil.

Hot-infused oil: Put 2 tsp powdered frank-incense resin and 1 cup grapeseed oil in a bowl; cover, and warm over a pan of simmering water for 2–3 hours. Cool, strain, bottle and store for up to 9 months.

259

Cedar of Lebanon *Cedrus libani*

The timber of this noble conifer has a dry spicy-wood aroma once enjoyed as incense by the Egyptians, Mesopotamians and Babylonians. Although now almost extinct, the tree still grows wild in Lebanon, where it is the national emblem. A cedar can sense the approach of snowfall and pre-emptively adjusts the curve of its branches to anticipate the weight of snow. It is therefore credited with the wisdom to understand the seasons and give eternal life. Herbalists use cedar of Lebanon to stem hair loss, as an expectorant to relieve chesty coughs, and to tone the skin. Test your skin sensitivity to its essential oil before using and avoid it altogether if you are pregnant.

Plant type:
Evergreen tree

Description: 30m (100ft) tall by 30m (100ft) wide; sweeping branches

Native habitat: Warm temperate; Lebanon, Turkey

Parts of plant used:
Wood, essential oil (from wood)

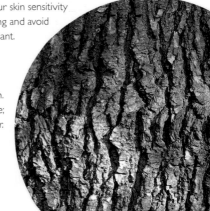

Growing and harvesting

- Grow in rich, well-drained, well-watered soil in full sun.
- Sow seeds in a greenhouse; leave there over the winter.
- Prune lower branches in spring. Dry these to make aromatic wood chips.

Lore and traditional uses

- In the Sumerian *Epic of Gilgamesh*, the home of the gods is the cedar forest of Lebanon.
- Since ancient times, cedar of Lebanon has been used in cosmetics and embalming, to cure leprosy and eliminate parasites.

Enhancing mind and spirit

- To create an uplifting, confidence-boosting space, vaporize 3 drops cedar of Lebanon essential oil in the room.
- To reduce emotional sensitivity, massage the neck and shoulders with cedar of Lebanon massage oil (see first preparation, right).

Caring for your body

- To encourage hair growth, massage 1–2 tsp cedar of Lebanon hair-loss oil (see second preparation, right) into the scalp, just before bed. Leave overnight, then wash out in the morning. Repeat daily for up to seven months.
- To tone the skin, add 4 drops of cedar of Lebanon essential oil to 30g (1oz) unscented skin cream and apply twice daily.

Core benefits

Boosts confidence

Promotes hair growth

Tones the skin

Preparations

Massage oil: Blend 2 drops each cedar of Lebanon and frankincense essential oils in 2 tsp sweet almond oil.

Hair-loss oil: Blend 3 drops each cedar of Lebanon, rosemary, lavender and thyme essential oils in ¼ cup sesame oil. Store in a sealed dark-glass jar for up to 6 months.

Myrrh *Commiphora myrrha*

According to the Gospel of Mark, myrrh resin mixed with wine was the intoxicant offered to Christ before he was crucified. As well as numbing the pain, the mix was believed to raise a person's spiritual state. Rich and woody with a hint of camphor, for centuries myrrh resin has been used for incense, perfume and embalming. It is steam-distilled to yield myrrh essential oil. When buying this oil, check that it is pure, without added ammonia, and avoid it during pregnancy. Herbalists use myrrh resin as an antiseptic for the throat, mouth and respiratory system and for its rejuvenating properties.

Plant type:
Shrub

Description: 5m (16ft) high by 5m (16ft) wide; thorny, scrubby, large shrub

Native habitat: Arid; Yemen, Somalia, Ethiopia, Kenya

Parts of plant used:
Resin, essential oil (from resin)

Growing and harvesting

- Prefers shallow soil over limestone, in full sun.
- Sow seeds in spring in a greenhouse.
- Resin exudes from bark fissures – make cuts in branches to increase resin production, then collect, and dry in the sun.

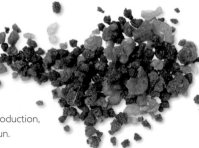

Lore and traditional uses

- The Chinese have used myrrh for 2,000 years as a wound-healer and blood-stimulant and Greek soldiers used it to treat battle wounds.
- Myrrh is a key ingredient in the Italian liqueur Fernet Branca, created as a medicine in 1845.

Enhancing mind and spirit

- To raise consciousness, with a sense of calm clarity, burn 1 tsp powdered myrrh resin on an incense disk while meditating (see p.253).
- To soothe anger or emotional pain, massage your body with 3 drops myrrh and 2 drops neroli essential oils in 2 tsp grapeseed oil.

Caring for your body

- To encourage cell renewal in wounds that are slow to heal, apply a little myrrh wound-healing blend (see first preparation, right) to the affected areas twice daily.
- To reduce inflamed gums, add 3 drops myrrh gum healer (see second preparation, right) to a glass of water; swish in the mouth for 2–3 minutes (then spit out) three times daily.

Core benefits

Raises consciousness

Heals the skin

Clears respiration

Preparations

Wound-healing blend: Mix 3 drops myrrh and 3 drops frankincense essential oils in 2 tsp sweet almond oil.

Gum healer: Mix 5 tsp myrrh tincture (200g/7oz powdered resin; standard method, p.20) with 1 tsp goldenseal tincture (see p.102), add 3 drops each tea tree and thyme and 10 drops peppermint essential oils; shake well.

Santang *Daniellia oliveri*

Each time I return to Gambia, I head for the market at Brikama to lose myself in the rich, enveloping balsam fragrance of santang. The resin is both cleansing and purging and the Gambians burn it to fumigate clothes and rooms and to expel disease-causing spirits. In the traditional medicine of West Africa, healers value the resin for its excellent antimicrobial, laxative and pain-relieving properties, using it as a skin soother, as a digestion aid and for its ability to treat headaches, toothache and menstrual pain. Its smoke deters mosquitoes. Avoid santang resin internally when pregnant.

Plant type:
Tree

Description: 30m (100ft) tall by 25m (80ft) wide; clusters of cream flowers

Native habitat: Tropical grassland; W Africa

Parts of plant used: Resin, bark, leaves, wood, roots, essential oil (from resin)

Growing and harvesting

- Grows in dry Tropics (sandy soil) with a rainy season.
- Easiest to cultivate from suckers; transplant and water until established, or sow seeds in greenhouse.
- Make a 20cm (8in) vertical cut in mature trunk. Scrape off collected resin, and dry.

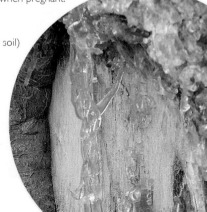

Lore and traditional uses

- Santang resin is used in West African religious ceremonies to raise spiritual consciousness.
- Timber from the santang tree is used to make drums, windowframes, furniture, beehives and quality charcoal; the resin is collected and moulded into "false" amber.

Enhancing mind and spirit

- To shed mental baggage, meditate on a theme of letting go, while burning ½ tsp powdered santang resin on an incense disk (see p.253).
- To create a protective aura around yourself, wear santang hot-infused oil (see first preparation, right) as a perfume.

Caring for your body

- To relieve itchy and inflamed skin, apply santang hot-infused oil (see first preparation, right) to the affected areas. (Check for skin sensitivity first.)
- To purge the body of toxins, drink 1 cup santang decoction (see second preparation, right), as required.

Core benefits

Lightens the spirit

Soothes the skin

Mosquito repellant

Preparations

Hot-infused oil: Put 1 tbsp crushed, dried santang resin and 1 cup grapeseed oil in a bowl over a pan of simmering water. Cover and leave for 2–3 hours. Cool, strain and store for up to 9 months.

Decoction: 30g (1oz) dried santang resin in 750ml (1½ pints) water. Standard method (p.20).

Juniper *Juniperus communis*

The juniper bush – which gives us the blue-black berries that flavour gin, Chartreuse liqueur and certain pâtés – is an aromatic conifer. The Babylonians, Egyptians and Tibetans burned its branches as a protective incense, while Native North Americans burned them in "sweat lodges" (dome-shaped huts for ritual purification) to cleanse the spirit of heavy emotional energies. In herbal medicine, juniper is a detoxifier and the berries' essential oil treats cellulite, cystitis, rheumatism, eczema and gout, and cleanses the emotions. Avoid the oil if you are pregnant or have kidney disease.

Plant type: Hardy, evergreen shrubby tree

Description: 10m (30ft) tall by 4m (13ft) wide; needle-like leaves

Native habitat: Cool temperate; Eurasia, N America

Part of plant used: Leaves, fruit, wood, essential oil (from fruit and twigs)

Growing and harvesting

- Prefers well-drained soil, in exposed sites in sun.
- Take 8cm (3in) mature-wood cuttings in autumn; plant in a greenhouse; need male and female trees for berries.
- Pick sprigs any time, then dry; pick berries when ripe in their second year, and dry.

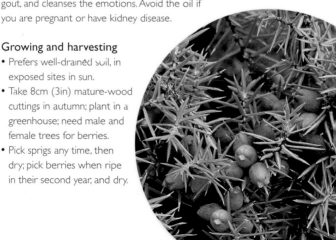

Lore and traditional uses

- Tibetan travellers burn juniper to ward off illnesses and to lift their prayers to heaven.
- Norwegians cook fresh fish on an outdoor grill covered with wet juniper branches, to give an instant smoked-juniper flavour.

Enhancing mind and spirit

- To cleanse the emotions and protect against negativity in a stressful environment, vaporize 3 drops juniper berry essential oil.
- To revitalize energy after strenuous activity, take a tepid bath laced with 6 drops juniper Viking oil blend (see first preparation, right).

Caring for your body

- To treat cellulite, use a skin brush over the affected areas (always sweep upward), then take a bath laced with 3 drops juniper berry and 3 drops rosemary essential oils. Massage the areas of cellulite under the water.
- To clear infection from the urinary tract, take 1 cup juniper berry infusion (see second preparation, right) twice daily, as needed.

Core benefits

Cleanses the spirit

Boosts energy

Diuretic

Preparations

Viking oil blend: Mix 10 drops each juniper berry, rosemary and black pepper essential oils and 5 drops peppermint essential oil.

Infusion: Steep 3 tsp dried juniper berries in 1 cup just-boiled water for 20 minutes. Strain, then drink.

267

Spikenard *Nardostachys jatamansi*

In India, this aromatic root – with a rich, musky fragrance – is used as incense to intensify spiritual devotion. The intense aroma is in the "collar" where the stem meets the root or rhizome and in the withered hair-like stems that are left when the leaves die. Various trials have confirmed that spikenard root collars have antifungal and antidepressant properties, help protect the liver and can increase levels of the body's mood-regulator, serotonin. The essential oil can promote the growth of hair and darken its colour.

Plant type:
Perennial

Description: 30cm (1ft) high by 20cm (8in) wide; pink–white flowers

Native habitat:
Mountain; Nepal, Bhutan

Parts of plant used:
Root collar

Growing and harvesting

- Prefers moisture-retentive soil in part shade.
- Transplant 20cm (8in) rhizome pieces in spring and water until well rooted. Or surface-sow ripe autumn seed (produced every three to four years) in a greenhouse, then plant out in late spring.
- Harvest root "collar" from two- to three-year-old plants; wash; dry in shade.

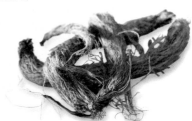

Lore and traditional uses

- Ayurvedic healers call spikenard the "divine plant", and prescribe it as a nerve tonic.
- Spikenard is an ancient culinary spice and featured in the recipe book of the Roman gourmet Apicius (1st century CE).

Enhancing mind and spirit

- To calm the mind and intensify spirituality, burn ½ tsp powdered spikenard root on an incense disk while meditating (see p.253).
- To balance the three *doshas* (see p.16), take 1 tsp spikenard tincture (see first preparation, right) three times daily.

Caring for the body

- To ease nerve-related headaches, and to help improve hair growth and colour, put 3 drops spikenard essential oil in 1 tsp sesame oil and massage into the scalp.
- To nourish mature skin, and to soothe away wrinkles, scars and rashes, apply spikenard face oil blend (see second preparation, right) every morning and evening.

Core benefits

Brings spirit into focus

Strengthens the mind

Soothes the nerves

Preparations

Tincture: 200g (7oz) dried or 400g (14oz) fresh, chopped spikenard root in 1 litre (2 pints) vodka-water mix. Standard method (p.20).

Face oil blend: Mix 3 drops spikenard and 3 drops lavender essential oils in 2 tsp grapeseed oil.

269

Copal *Protium copal*

I have a tiny woven bag from Guatemala that hangs on my kitchen door; inside are pine needles, wood chips and a piece of copal resin – for protection. The resin has a warm, hypnotic, woody fragrance, and since the times of the ancient Aztecs and Maya, Central Americans have considered it protective and purifying. Generically, the term copal is used to describe the pliable halfway point between a liquid resin and hard nuggets. Copal is sold as three types: "white", which has a light and fruity scent; "gold", which is rich and smooth; and "black", which is deep and mysterious. Used therapeutically, the resin can improve dental and respiratory health, and the bark can eliminate intestinal parasites.

Plant type:
Evergreen tree

Description: 10m (30ft) tall by 8m (25ft) wide; red fruit

Native habitat: Tropical rainforest; C America

Parts of plant used: Resin, bark, essential oil (from resin)

Growing and harvesting

- Prefers well-drained, sandy soil with high humidity and shade.
- Sow ripe seed in a greenhouse. Or take flexible cuttings in spring.
- Drill small holes in the bark of mature trees to harvest resin; dry.

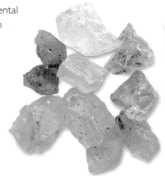

Lore and traditional uses

- Central American shamans inhaled the smoke of copal resin, along with other substances, to achieve trance-like states.
- Mayans considered copal to be nature's food for the gods. They believed the resin should never be touched by hand, so used special tools when placing it on an altar.

Enhancing the spirit

- To relieve tension and calm the mind, massage the body with copal hot-infused oil (see first preparation, right), as required.
- To protect a room from negativity, place ½ tsp powdered copal resin on each of four incense disks. Light the powder and place the disks in the corners of the room (see p.253).

Caring for your body

- To relieve indigestion caused by a nervous stomach, apply a copal hot compress (see second preparation, right) as hot as tolerable to your abdomen. Rest with the compress in place for as long as is comfortable.

Core benefits

Protects the spirit

Soothes the nerves

Aids digestion

Preparations

Hot-infused oil: Put 1 tbsp crushed dried copal resin and 1 cup grapeseed oil in a bowl over a pan of simmering water. Cover and leave for 2–3 hours. Cool and strain. Store for up to 9 months.

Hot compress: Put 4–6 drops copal essential oil in a bowl of just-boiled water. Soak a flannel in the water.

Clary sage *Salvia sclarea*

Clary sage has tall, flowering stems of dusty pinks and subtle mauves – all with a haunting pungency. Each individual will find that the herb's effects are remarkably attuned to his or her own circumstances – its effects can be anything from mildly inebriating to spiritually uplifting, depending upon your state of mind or needs at the time. The herb has a strong effect on the female hormones, so avoid it during pregnancy. Avoid taking it with alcohol, too.

Plant type:
Hardy biennial

Description: 1.5m (5ft) high by 1m (3ft) wide; mauve and pink flowers

Native habitat: All temperate; Europe, C Asia

Parts of plant used: Flowers, leaves, seeds, essential oil (from flowering tops)

Growing and harvesting
- Grows in well-drained, sandy soil in sun; it dislikes wet winters.
- Sow seeds in spring or summer (the plant will self-seed).
- Harvest leaves and flowering tops as needed; harvest seeds when ripe in early autumn. Use fresh, or dry.

Lore and traditional uses
- In Germany, clary sage was sometimes used by wine

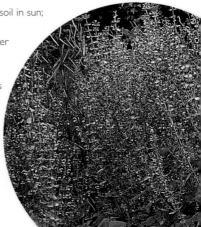

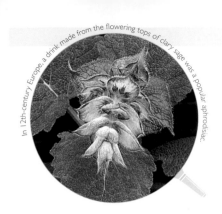

In 12th-century Europe, a drink made from the flowering tops of clary sage was a popular aphrodisiac.

Core benefits

Spiritual awakener

Enhances dream recall

Eases menopause

merchants to enchance the characteristic musky aroma of Muscatel wines.

Enhancing the spirit

- To improve dream recall and to take spiritual lessons from your subconscious, put 1 drop clary sage essential oil on your pillow.

Caring for your body

- To relieve menopause symptoms, take 1 cup clary sage infusion (see first preparation, right) three times daily, until symptoms ease.
- To dislodge debris from the eyes, and clarify and refresh them, apply clary sage soaked seed treatment (see second preparation, right), using a sterile eye cup for each eye.

Preparations

Infusion: 2 tsp fresh or dry clary sage leaves or flowering tops in 1 cup just-boiled water. Standard method (p.20).

Soaked seed treatment: Just cover 50–100g (1¾–3½oz) clary sage seeds with water. Soak overnight or until seeds are soft. Strain the seed mucilage and use it immediately.

Sandalwood *Santalum album*

Walking down Mount Putou in China 20 years ago, I suddenly became aware of the scent of sandalwood. Drawn toward the fresh, green fragrance, I discovered monks rebuilding a Taoist temple using this rare wood – the traditional material for temple structures. Sandalwood's sapwood provides a meditation aid in all major religions. The essential oil comes primarily from the tree's heartwood and roots, and is used to soothe tension and moisturize dry, cracked and mature skin. It is also an antiseptic for the lungs and urinary tract, and an aphrodisiac.

Plant type:
Evergreen tree

Description: 18m (60ft) tall by 10m (30ft) wide; yellow-to-purple flowers

Native habitat: Tropical grassland; SE Asia

Parts of plant used:
Whole tree (including roots), essential oil (from heartwood)

Growing and harvesting

- Requires well-drained soil; long, dry periods; plentiful sun, but cool air.
- Grow from root suckers. Or sow ripe seeds 2cm (¾in) deep along with capsicum as a "host" plant; water lightly. When 1–2m (3–7ft) tall, move to a permanent site next to a larger host, such as *Acacia* or *Vitex* species.

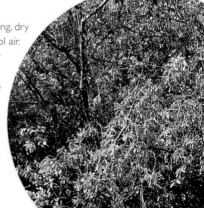

- Whole trees are harvested into wood chips only once they are 40 years old or more.

Lore and traditional uses
- In India, sandalwood is used for funeral pyres to protect the soul's onward spiritual passage from the influence of evil spirits.
- Hindus traditionally use coloured sandalwood paste to create the *bindi* forehead dot, to bring a closer connection to the divine.

Enhancing mind and spirit
- To awaken spiritual intelligence, meditate while burning ½ tsp sandalwood powder on an incense disk (see p.253).

Caring for the body
- To moisturize dry, split skin on the heels, massage nightly with sandalwood cracked heel blend (see first preparation, right).
- To clear an infection in the urinary tract, take 1 tsp sandalwood tincture (see second preparation, right) three or four times daily, until the infection has gone.

Core benefits
Calms the mind

Replenishes the skin

Antiseptic

Preparations

Cracked heel blend: Mix together 3 drops each sandalwood and lavender essential oils in 2 tbsp infused calendula flower oil (see p.23). Seal, then store (use within 9 months).

Tincture: 200g (7oz) dried sandalwood bark chips or powder in 1 litre (2 pints) vodka-water mix. Standard method (p.20).

Glossary

aerial parts parts of a plant that live above the ground, including the stem, leaves and flowers

alluvial soil that is rich with a mixture of clay, silt and sand

antioxidant a compound that prevents oxidization of cells, and so inhibits the action of **free radicals**

astringent a substance that causes the body's cells to contract and tighten

carrier oil natural, vegetable oil used to dilute **essential oils** so they can be applied to the skin

climate the weather conditions for a particular region. The climate in which you live determines which plants you can grow most easily, and whether you need to grow certain plants inside (say, in a greenhouse), and at what stage of growing and times of year you can put plants outside in a soil bed. I have divided the world into seven climate systems based on modern geographical zones. These appear under the "Native habitat" for each plant in the guide

• **arid** dry, often desert, regions with very low annual rainfall

• **coniferous forest** (also called taiga) regions of the north Northern hemisphere that are cold all year

• **cool temperate** cooler regions, mostly in the Northern hemisphere, although also in parts of southeast Asia and in New Zealand, with high rainfall at certain seasons

• **mountain** regions, such as the Andes, Himalaya and Rockies, 3,000m (10,000ft) or more above sea level

• **tropical grassland** hot, tropical regions, such as the savanna, with some summer rain

• **tropical rainforest** hot, tropical regions, with rain all year

• **warm temperate** warmer regions with low rainfall, mostly comprising the Mediterranean regions of southern Europe and north Africa, and parts of the USA and southern Australia

cold frame small, boxed enclosure with a glass lid used to protect plants from cold weather conditions, or acclimatize plants that have been grown in a greenhouse before planting outside

corm bulb-like swelling at the base of the

stem of certain plants (such as crocus), which can produce new plants

cutting a piece cut from a mature plant and used to propagate new plants

emollient a preparation that softens, moisturizes and soothes the skin

expectorant a preparation that encourages the body to expel mucus from the respiratory system

essential oil the volatile oil in certain plant cells, giving a plant its aroma

flowering top the very top of a stem that produces buds that flower

frame metal or wooden structure used to support plants with weak stems, as in climbers and some bushy perennials

free radicals unstable molecules that oxidize cells in the body, damaging them and potentially causing cancer

hand hot hot to touch, but not scolding

heel the swollen piece of a main stem at the junction with a side stem

host plant the plant on which another plant lives or feeds

humus-rich type of soil enriched with decomposed leaves and other organic plant material

loamy type of soil made up of clay, sand and **humus**; it holds moisture well, but

drains any excess

mist chamber small enclosure containing a misting device that leaves a film of moisture on the **aerial parts** of a plant

mucilage a viscous or gelatinous plant secretion (such as from the roots or seeds), often with soothing properties

offset side growth from the base of a biennial or perennial capable of becoming a new plant

pinch out to take off the growing tip of a main or side stem

plant out to move a growing plant from inside, perhaps in a greenhouse, to outside in a soil bed, usually in stages so the plant can acclimatize

rhizome the horizontal, underground, root-producing stem of certain plants

rootstock shortened stem of a shrub or tree onto which plants may be grafted

runner (similar to **rhizome**) plant shoot that grows at the base of a stem along the ground; it can root at any point along its length

side shoot side branch or stem, or secondary stem

sucker a shrub or tree shoot growing from the base of the stem or from the roots, capable of becoming a new plant **277**

Bibliography

Abbiw, Daniel K., *Useful Plants of Ghana* Royal Botanic Gardens, Kew (London, UK), 1990

Bremness, Lesley, *The Complete Book of Herbs*, Dorling Kindersley in Association with the National Trust (London, UK), 1988

Bremness, Lesley, *Crabtree & Evelyn Fragrant Herbal*, Quadrille Publishing (London, UK), 1998

Bremness, Lesley, *Eyewitness Handbook of Herbs: 700 Species from Around the World*, Dorling Kindersley (London, UK), 1994, updated 2000

Chevallier, Andrew, *The Encyclopedia of Medicinal Plants*, Dorling Kindersley (London, UK), 1996

China Health Committee, Hunan Province, *A Barefoot Doctor's Manual*, Cloudburst Press (Seattle, USA), 1977

Davis, Patricia, *Subtle Aromatherapy*, C.W. Daniel (Saffron Walden, UK), 1991

Fu Weikang, *Traditional Chinese Medicine and Pharmacology*, Foreign Language Press (Beijing, China), 1985

Genders, Roy, *Scented Flora of the World*, Robert Hale (London, UK), 1977

Graves, Robert, *The White Goddess*, Faber and Faber (London, UK), 1961

Gurudas, *Flower Essences*, Brotherhood of Life (Albuquerque, New Mexico, USA), 1983

Kaptchuk, Ted, *The Web That Has No Weaver; Understanding Chinese Medicine*, Thomas Nelson (Ontario, Canada), 1983

Lawless, Julia, *The Illustrated Encyclopedia of Essential Oils*, Element (London, UK), 1995

Thistleton-Dyer, W.T., *The Folk-Lore of Plants*, Appleton (New York, USA), 1889

Tompkins, Peter and Bird, Christopher, *The Secret Life of Plants*, Avon Books (New York, USA), 1973

Valnet, Dr Jean, *The Practice of Aromatherapy*, C.W. Daniel (Saffron Walden, UK), 1982

Warrier, Gopi and Gunawant, Deepika MD, *Ayurveda*, Element (London, UK), 1997

Index

Picture credits

The publisher would like to thank the following organizations, photographers and photographic libraries for permission to reproduce their material. Every care has been taken to trace copyright holders. However, if we have omitted anyone, we apologize and will, if informed, make corrections to any future edition.

Deni Bown: 1, 2, 5 left, centre, right; 8, 46, 49 left, centre; 50, 58, 60, 61, 64, 66, 69, 71 left, centre, right; 72, 75, 76, 78, 81, 82, 83, 84, 86, 87, 89, 91 left, centre, right; 92, 94, 98, 100, 103, 105, 106, 109, 113 left, centre, right; 114, 117, 118, 120, 122, 123, 125, 126, 129, 132, 134, 137 centre, right; 138, 140, 144, 146, 150, 154, 162, 164, 169 left, centre, right; 170, 172, 173, 175, 176, 179, 180, 184, 185, 186, 188, 193 left, centre, right; 194, 196, 198, 200, 203, 204, 207, 212, 215, 216, 219, 220, 221, 223 left, centre, right; 224, 226, 228, 230, 232, 233, 234, 237, 238, 242, 244, 246, 247, 253 left, centre, right; 256, 258, 266, 272, 274.

Bodleian Library, University of Oxford/MS.Bodl. 130, fol. 56r:12; British Library/Art Archive:16; British Library/akg:19; Koichi Saito/Corbis: 21; Lou Chardonnay/Corbis: 22; Imagemore/Corbis: 25; Sharie Kennedy/Corbis: 28; Verity Welstead/Getty: 31; Steven Mark Needham/Corbis: 33; Tim McConville/Corbis: 34; Clay Perry/Corbis: 37; Imagewerks/Getty: 44; George Diebold/Getty: 49, 56; Duncan Baird Archive: 52, 54, 68, 99, 190, 268; Iata Cannabrava/Getty: 63; Imagemore/Getty: 96; Geoff Kidd/Science Photolibrary: 110, 182, 250; TH Foto-Werberg/Photolibrary: 119; FhfGreenmedia/ GAP Photos: 131; Janet Seaton/Photolibrary: 137 left, 166; Lesley Bremness: 142, 264; Siri Stafford/Getty: 147; Jovan Denberg/Stockfood: 149, 153; Howard Rice/ Photolibrary: 156; Maximillian Stock/Science Photolibrary: 158; Bob Gibbons/Science Photolibrary:160; Eberhart Wally/Photolibrary: 208; Flowerphotos: 210; Dave King/ Stockfood: 240; Bildagentur/Science Photolibrary: 248; Neil Fletcher & Matthew Ward/DK Images: 254, 270; Dennis Flaherty/Science Photolibrary: 257; C.Sappa/ Getty: 260; Neil Fletcher & Matthew Ward/Getty: 262

Useful websites

The following organizations can provide helpful information on where to buy and how to use herbs:

In the UK: www.herbsociety.org.uk
In the USA: www.herbsociety.org
In Canada: www.herbsocietymb.com
In Australia: www.allrareherbs.com.au

Acknowledgments

Author's acknowledgments: A big bouquet to DBP for two wonderful editors – Joanna Micklem and Judy Barratt – for keeping the book's vision of wholeness with the right balance of cajoling praise and dutiful discipline, and especially to Judy for sharing late-night emails with unfailing good humour. Plus, a quick bow to the man behind "Bob's Angels", and to designer Daniel Sturges for producing sterling work amid multitudinous extra requests. An enormous thank you to my colleague Walter Enns, a Master Herbalist of 35 years who advised on our herbal prescriptions for mind and body. A most welcome research-assistant manifest in the form of number-three son, J.J. Lowe, also a writer, who helped make the wide scope of subjects in this book possible in the available time. And always thanks for the support of all my sons. For this book I had the opportunity to meet more herbal trees and shrubs in Africa, thanks to Mr Jerreh Touray of Gambia.

Finally, I dedicate this book to the memory of my sister Dr Adrienne Wendy May Bremness, Shiatsu master, nutritionist, healer of animals, doctor of Oriental Medicine (99.8% in her exam!), Chinese Herbs and Acupuncture. A life well lived.

Publisher's acknowledgments: The publisher would like to thank Master Herbalist Walter Enns for his invaluable help, and Deni Bown for her advice and photographs.

CHAPTER 1

Invigorators and Stimulants

Every time your body, mind or spirit needs a boost, turn to these zesty tonics. This chapter presents a wealth of refreshing, stimulating herbs that will rouse your system in the morning and provide spirited pick-me-ups at any other time of day.

Among the most invigorating are common herbs such as cool, clean peppermint (indeed the whole mint family), as well as lesser-known plants, such as alecost, which has sharp, tangy leaves and an energizing, minty scent with an added hint of spice.

The sun-kissed citrus family features here, too. Think how pleasing and uplifting it can be when someone peels an orange on a crowded train; or how refreshing it is to drink a cold glass of homemade lemonade on a hot afternoon.

One of the most unusual herbs to appear in this chapter is the South American herb guaraná, the seeds of which